T0091575

Failure to Thrive
and Malnutrition

Joyee Goswami Vachani
Editor

Failure to Thrive and Malnutrition

A Practical, Evidence-Based
Clinical Guide

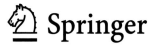 Springer

Editor
Joyee Goswami Vachani
Baylor College of Medicine/ Texas Children's Hospital
Houston, TX, USA

ISBN 978-3-031-14163-8   ISBN 978-3-031-14164-5   (eBook)
https://doi.org/10.1007/978-3-031-14164-5

This Springer imprint is published by the registered company Springer Nature Switzerland AG
The registered company address is: Gewerbestrasse 11, 6330 Cham, Switzerland

Preface

As a pediatrician who strives to continually integrate evidence-based medicine into practice, I have always been intrigued with failure to thrive (FTT). FTT is often a multifactorial diagnosis requiring multidisciplinary treatment, making a precise definition difficult. Historical definitions (organic vs. nonorganic, crossing percentiles) often do not capture the complex interaction among a child's medical, nutritional, and social/environmental needs. While some studies are shifting towards using the term growth faltering to describe forms of undernutrition, we use the term failure to thrive for this book.

This book aims to review current evidence in diagnostic and management strategies for failure to thrive. By applying evidence in the literature on the following topics, we intend to give practitioners a systematic approach they can integrate into practice.

- Definition
- Differential diagnosis
- Growth assessment
- Management approach—enteral nutrition
- Management approach—the importance of a multi-disciplinary
- Impact of social determinants of health/health disparities
- Improvement opportunities including insight on developing a clinical pathway

One of the challenges in writing this book is the constantly changing landscape and impact of both the pandemic and local/national policies. Food insecurity is a well-described factor which continues to increase and directly impacts children with FTT and their families. I appreciate the hard work of all the authors in this dynamic environment and would like to thank each of them for their dedication and expertise in contributing to this book and field of work. I would also like to thank my family, friends, and the children/families we have the privilege and honor to care for—they are truly our continuous source of inspiration.

Houston, TX   Joyee Goswami Vachani

Contents

Chapter 1
Definition

Margaret S. Wood

Background

Healthy infancy and childhood are marked by growth and development. Newborns require specific environmental conditions to grow and develop. The connection between growth and nutrition occupies a large portion of parent and provider attention. Parents may find themselves confused or frustrated by the processes involved in breastfeeding a newborn. Latching, positioning, and nursing do not always come naturally. Mixing formula and assembling bottles can be a difficult task. Each family must learn to respond to their individual child's needs and cues. As every child has a unique growth trajectory and potential, it is standard of care for pediatric providers to plot each child on a standardized growth chart and monitor for deviations. Because growth and development involve a complex process of biology, environment, and society, it is important to investigate further when evaluating and treating children for concerns of failure to thrive.

M. S. Wood (✉)
Department of Pediatrics, Baylor College of Medicine, Texas Children's Hospital, Houston, TX, USA
e-mail: mswood1@texaschildrens.org

© Springer Nature Switzerland AG 2023   1
J. G. Vachani (ed.), *Failure to Thrive and Malnutrition*,
https://doi.org/10.1007/978-3-031-14164-5_1

History

Historically many different terms have been used to describe the specific syndrome referred to as failure to thrive (FTT). Some of the first descriptions in the medical literature were in the 1960s when FTT was referred to as a "syndrome of maternal deprivation" [1]. This definition focused on the interplay of various factors involved in the lack of expected growth of the child, not just inadequate nutrition. Early case presentations included detailed growth charts demonstrating inappropriately low weight gain over time. These case histories also described both the anthropomorphic measurements of the parents and included psychosocial assessments. Mothers predominantly would be described by age, educational attainment, employment, marital status, and affect. The mother's attitude toward the affected child and the concept of motherhood as a developmental phase were often detailed [2]. Literature in the 1970s described failure to thrive as "weight faltering," "feeding problems" indicative of a "stressful mother-child relationship," and a "deprivation syndrome" [3].

These historical language choices are outdated but did help characterize the clinical presentation of FTT as encompassing a spectrum of clinical findings, with unclear or complex etiology and not simply malnutrition. Failure to thrive as a clinical syndrome distinct from malnutrition is predicated predominantly on access to food. The definition of FTT required language developed to describe a child who, without obvious or overt starvation, was not growing adequately or in some cases was actually losing weight. As such, further descriptions attempted to divide this syndrome into subcategories. Much of the subsequent language in medical literature distinguished "organic" as opposed to "non-organic" or "psychosocial" failure to thrive [4–6]. This distinction in terminology pointed clinicians toward the task of identifying differences in etiology and thus the need for different therapeutic approaches. Given a specific clinical presentation— history taking, physical examination, and laboratory testing were guided by a desire to uncover medical pathology or familial/social factors as key drivers of a child's faltering growth.

Description

Merriam Webster's Collegiate dictionary defines the word "thrive" as "to grow vigorously" with "flourish" as a synonym. More eloquently, "to progress toward or realize a goal despite or because of circumstances" [7]. In this understanding, thriving encompasses more than just mere weight gain or objective growth, but also points to a broad type of progress encompassing the environment of the child. In this context, a child who fails to thrive lacks vigor in growth and fails to progress to a goal.

Because the clinical state of the child who was failing to grow was so intertwined with the child's environment and primary parental relationship, descriptions focused on subjective understandings of parent–child connection and family situations [1]. These terms spoke to the broader failure of expected normal growth and development in the absence of an obvious cause. As time progressed, the term failure to thrive came more into common use and avoids explicitly pejorative language about parenting, and specifically mothering. The term failure to thrive is also a more accurate description of a broad problem with the implied potential for multiple causes [8]. In current literature, failure to thrive can alternatively be referred to as "growth faltering," "weight faltering," or "poor weight gain"—descriptive of symptoms of undernutrition [9].

Growth Charts

To understand when an infant or child's growth deviates from what is normal or would be expected requires an understanding of what *is* normal or expected. To that end, public health organizations have created standard growth charts to be used as references for normal development. By compiling the measurements from a very large sample of infants and children, statistical techniques can create an expression of median measurements and their change over time. An individual clinician can then use these growth charts to compare a child's growth to what could be expected of a typical child from a given population. Historically, growth charts have included weight and some combination of length or height as well as head circumference.

In the United States, the first national growth charts were developed in 1977 by the Centers for Disease Control and Prevention [10]. These charts were widely adopted as a reference standard for child growth and also used outside the United States through dissemination by the World Health Organization [10]. The original 1977 growth charts were based off of a small population of children from a limited geographic area in the state of Ohio. The measurement data used to create these charts was drawn from National Health and Nutrition Examination Survey (NHANES). These children were mostly fed via formula as was typical for children in the United States at that time [10].

Observational studies indicate infants who are predominantly fed with formula display different growth patterns in infancy compared to babies who are breastfed. Specifically, infants fed formula show increased rates of weight gain compared to exclusively breastfed babies [11, 12].

In response to concerns that the original 1977 CDC growth charts were not representative of and/or relevant for general pediatric populations, the CDC published revised charts in 2000 [10]. These growth charts used statistical techniques to mark lines of weight for age, length or height for age, head circumference for age, weight for length or height, and body mass index (BMI). These charts have lines to demarcate growth percentiles for age, with the median being marked with the 50th percentile line.

To use these growth curves, the intersection between a child's age on the horizontal axis and a child's measured size on the vertical axis is marked. Over time, subsequent measurements can also be marked and a line drawn between them to demonstrate a child's individual growth trajectory. This is compared to the closest percentile line on the chart to estimate a child's individual growth percentile for age.

A child's expressed percentile for age on the chart refers to the percent of children in the sample population who would be expected to have a smaller measurement than the child. Today, many electronic medical records software will automatically plot a child's measurements from recorded vital signs. The software may also calculate a specific percentile and graph the child's growth trajectory over time. This is a useful way to both visually and mathematically see a child's individual measurements compared to a reference population [10, 13].

Oftentimes growth parameters are expressed as a percentile for age, or a z-score. The z-score is a statistical term that refers to the calculation of a child's difference from the mean measurement for a child of the same age in the reference population, divided by the standard deviation of that measurement in the reference population. A calculated z-score would be positive if a child measures larger than the mean and is a negative value if the child measures smaller than the mean. Because they are both mathematical calculations, percentile for age, and z-score for age express the same concept: the 97th percentile for age on a given growth curve corresponds to a z-score of 1.88 and a z-score of negative 1.88 corresponds to a measurement at the third percentile for age. The CDC does caution that due to the statistical methods used and the population size of the sample, the growth curves are not meant to be used to extrapolate percentiles outside of two standard deviations (the third percentile up to the 97th percentile) [10, 13].

While the CDC growth charts were initially used internationally, the WHO developed and released its own growth charts in 2006 [13]. The WHO growth charts were created from the data collected from the WHO Multicentre Growth Reference Study (MGRS) [14]. This study collected measurements from infants and children from six countries: Brazil, Ghana, India, Norway, Oman, and the United States. The study employed a methodology designed to select healthy children with nonsmoking mothers in an effort to capture the true genetic potential for growth without environmental deprivation. Subjects also were selected using an assumption of breastfeeding being the "biological norm" for infants [13, 14]. All the children in the studied population were breastfed for at least 12 months and most were exclusively breastfed for at least the first 4 months of life [13–15]. Measurements were collected over time from infants up until 2 years of age and cross-sectional measurements from samples of children 18–71 months of age [16]. WHO growth charts display the weight for age measurements from birth to 5 years of age, length for age measurements from birth to 24 months of age, and height for age measurements from 2 to 5 years of age. They also include calculated weight for length, weight for height, and body mass index for age [13].

In 2010, the CDC recommended the WHO growth charts be used to plot children's growth under 2 years of age and that the CDC growth charts be used for children over 2 years of age in the United States [15]. This is based on the understanding that the WHO growth charts are representative of a more diverse population both nutritionally and genetically.

With the shift from CDC growth chart measurements to WHO charts, observational studies have shown differing incidences in diagnosis of failure to thrive [17]. It is also important to understand that growth charts are created from averages of large groups of children, and each individual child will not always follow an exact percentile of the curve or stay a similar distance to the median throughout childhood. Especially in the first year of life studies show that many children cross one or more growth percentiles both up and down [16, 18].

In more recent years, growth curves have been created to characterize the normal weight loss trajectory and recovery in the first hours, days, and weeks of an infant's life [19–21]. With technology, an individual newborn's hour-by-hour weight loss or gain can be mapped onto a curve created based on healthy, breastfed babies born in the United States. Analogously to how the risk of severe jaundice and kernicterus is predicted based on hour-by-hour measurements of serum bilirubin, a newborn's hourly weight can be used to identify early problems with weight loss, slow weight gain, or to reassure families that a given degree of weight loss is typical compared to other infants.

Nutrition

The consensus statement of the Academy of Nutrition and Dietetics/American Society for Parenteral and Enteral Nutrition recommends that undernutrition be identified in a number of different ways depending on the availability of measurement techniques and time. If only one point in time of measurement is used, they recommend that undernutrition be defined by z-score of weight for height, body mass index (BMI) percentile for age, length or height for age, or mid-upper arm circumference (MUAC) [22]. The mid-upper arm circumference is an especially useful measurement in areas where equipment for height and weight are not available as a measuring tape is easily mobile.

When two or more measurements over time are available for a given child, a deceleration of weight for height z-score can be used to identify children with undernutrition. The weight gain velocity can be calculated for children under 2 years old and for children over 2 years old weight loss can be similarly used as an identifier of undernutrition. If multiple encounters have occurred with a child over time, an objective log of the nutritional intake can be an important component of the clinical picture.

The malnutrition literature has also come to measure the degree of undernutrition and created objective definitions for mild, moderate, and severe malnutrition. Mild malnutrition is defined as a z-score of −1 to −1.9, moderate malnutrition as z-score − 2 to −2.9, and severe malnutrition as z-score less than −3 [22].

Definition

The history of the identification and definition of failure to thrive as a clinical syndrome is broad. It encompasses a degree of negative deviation either in absolute measurement or in decreasing velocity of growth over time as expected for a child. Failure to thrive also requires further investigation to elicit a potential underlying cause. Consensus exists that failure to thrive can be inferred from a single absolute growth measurement that would meet malnutrition criteria (more than 2 standard deviations from the median or less than the third percentile for age). Failure to thrive can also be inferred when a child demonstrates a decline in growth velocity over time, which can be characterized by the crossing of multiple growth percentiles [5, 9, 23].

These objective measurements alone, however, do not encompass all that is meant by the broader term of failure to thrive. A child may have a weight for height z-score of −3 during a famine and while that meets the criteria for failure to thrive, it would be more appropriate and specific to diagnose that child as having severe acute malnutrition due to inadequate diet. In contrast, a child with failure to thrive — when we are speaking of failure to thrive as a diagnostic dilemma — may not have an immediate, clear cause [23]. To fail to thrive means both too-small measurements and the lack of expected flourishing and fulfillment of potential for a child [8, 23, 24].

Medical Coding

In the medical coding system, failure to thrive as a clinical syndrome does qualify as a reimbursable code. Before 2015, the United States used the ICD 9 codes that categorize failure to thrive as 783.41 — failure to thrive in a child, 779.34 — failure to thrive in an infant less than 28 days, or 783.7 — failure to thrive in an adult. Since 2015, the ICD 10 codes listed below have been used [25, 26]. Coding the degree of malnutrition allows for a more complete picture so it is important to include this information when available.

• FTT	R62.51
• FTT in newborn	P92.6
• Feeding difficulties and mismanagement	R63.3
• Feeding problems in newborn	P92
• Loss of weight	R63.4
• Malnutrition of moderate degree	E44.0
• Malnutrition, unspecified	E46
• Nutritional deficiency, unspecified	E63.9
• Underweight	R63.6

References

1. Patton RG, Gardner LI. Influence of family environment on growth: the syndrome of "maternal deprivation". Pediatrics. 1962;30(6):957–62.
2. Leonard MF, Rhymes JP, Solnit AJ. Failure to thrive in infants: a family problem. Am J Dis Child. 1966;111(6):600–12.
3. Hannaway PJ. Failure to thrive: a study of 100 infants and children. Clin Pediatr. 1970;9(2):96–9.
4. Berwick DM. Nonorganic failure-to-thrive. Pediatr Rev. 1980;1(9):265–70.
5. Jaffe AC. Failure to thrive: current clinical concepts. Pediatr Rev. 2011;32(3):100–7. quiz 108
6. Sills RH. Failure to thrive: the role of clinical and laboratory evaluation. Am J Dis Child. 1978;132(10):967–9.
7. Staff M. Merriam-Webster's collegiate dictionary. Merriam-Webster; 2004.
8. Marcovitch H. Fortnightly reviews: failure to thrive. BMJ. 1994;308(6920):35.

9. Tang MN, Adolphe S, Rogers SR, Frank DA. Failure to thrive or growth faltering: medical, developmental/behavioral, nutritional, and social dimensions. Pediatr Rev. 2021;42(11):590–603.

10. Kuczmarski RJ. 2000 CDC Growth Charts for the United States: methods and development. Department of Health and Human Services, Centers for Disease Control and ...; 2002.

11. Bell KA, Wagner CL, Feldman HA, Shypailo RJ, Belfort MB. Associations of infant feeding with trajectories of body composition and growth. Am J Clin Nutr. 2017;106(2):491–8.

12. Dewey KG. Growth characteristics of breast-fed compared to formula-fed infants. Biol Neonate. 1998;74(2):94–105.

13. World Health Organization. WHO child growth standards: length/height-for-age, weight-for-age, weight-for-length, weight-for-height and body mass index-for-age: methods and development. 2006.

14. De Onis M, Garza C, Victora CG, Onyango AW, Frongillo EA, Martines J. The WHO Multicentre Growth Reference Study: planning, study design, and methodology. Food Nutr Bull. 2004;25(1_suppl_1):S15–26.

15. Grummer-Strawn LM, Reinold C, Krebs NF, Centers for Disease Control and Prevention (CDC). Use of World Health Organization and CDC growth charts for children aged 0–59 months in the United States. MMWR Recomm Rep. 2010;59(RR-9):1–15.

16. Bennett WE Jr, Hendrix KS, Thompson RT, Carroll AE, Downs SM. The natural history of weight percentile changes in the first year of life. JAMA Pediatr. 2014;168(7):681–2.

17. Daymont C, Hoffman N, Schaefer EW, Fiks AG. Clinician diagnoses of failure to thrive before and after switch to World Health Organization Growth curves. Acad Pediatr. 2019;20(3):405–12.

18. Mei Z, Grummer-Strawn LM, Thompson D, Dietz WH. Shifts in percentiles of growth during early childhood: analysis of longitudinal data from the California Child Health and Development Study. Pediatrics. 2004;113(6):e617–27.

19. Flaherman VJ, Schaefer EW, Kuzniewicz MW, Li SX, Walsh EM, Paul IM. Early weight loss nomograms for exclusively breastfed newborns. Pediatrics. 2015;135(1):e16–23.

20. Paul IM, Schaefer EW, Miller JR, Kuzniewicz MW, Li SX, Walsh EM, et al. Weight change nomograms for the first month after birth. Pediatrics. 2016;138(6):e20162625. https://doi.org/10.1542/peds.2016-2625.

21. Schaefer EW, Flaherman VJ, Kuzniewicz MW, Li SX, Walsh EM, Paul IM. External validation of early weight loss nomograms for exclusively breastfed newborns. Breastfeed Med. 2015;10(10):458–63.
22. Becker P, Carney LN, Corkins MR, Monczka J, Smith E, Smith SE, et al. Consensus statement of the Academy of Nutrition and Dietetics/American Society for Parenteral and Enteral Nutrition: indicators recommended for the identification and documentation of pediatric malnutrition (undernutrition). Nutr Clin Pract. 2015;30(1):147–61.
23. Larson-Nath C, Biank VF. Clinical review of failure to thrive in pediatric patients. Pediatr Ann. 2016;45(2):e46–9.
24. Donaldson M. Failure to thrive: define it carefully. BMJ. 1994;308(6928):596.
25. Centers for Medicare and Medicaid Services. Overview: ICD-10. 2019. Available at: https://www.cms.gov/Medicare/Coding/ICD10. Accessed 30 Jan 2020.
26. Linzer JF. Pediatric code crosswalk ICD-9-cm to ICD-10-cm. Elk Grove Village, IL: American Academy of Pediatrics; 2013.

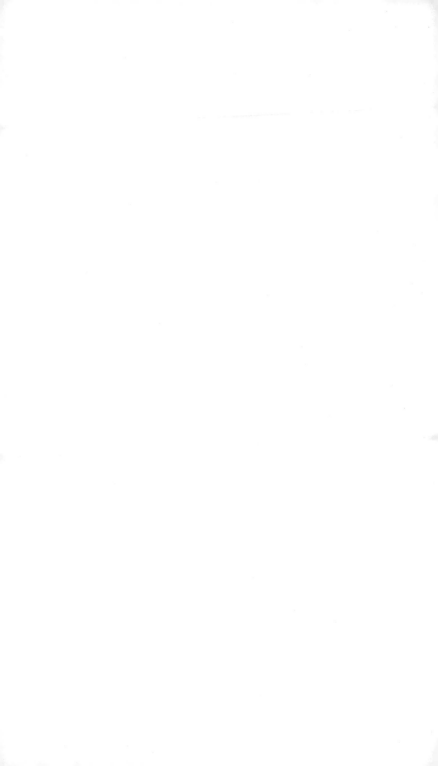

Chapter 2
Differential Diagnosis of Failure to Thrive

Fatima Gutierrez and Aldo Maspons

Approach to Differential of Patient with Failure to Thrive

The historical classification of failure to thrive as organic versus nonorganic is no longer valid as failure to thrive is a multifactorial process often involving both biological and social factors. Weight gain and weight loss are a function of calories so patients with failure to thrive can be categorized in three main areas: (1) not enough calories in, (2) too many calories out (loss of calories), and (3) need for more calories (an increased metabolic demand). Although the differential diagnosis of failure to thrive also varies by age, the approach is the same.

History and physical exam are fundamental components in developing a differential diagnosis in a patient with failure to thrive. Key elements in history taking include details

F. Gutierrez (✉)
Department of Pediatrics, Texas Tech University Health Sciences Center, El Paso, TX, USA
e-mail: Fatima.gutierrez@ttuhsc.edu

A. Maspons
Maspons Pediatric Gastro LLC, El Paso, TX, USA
e-mail: aldo@drmaspons.com

© Springer Nature Switzerland AG 2023
J. G. Vachani (ed.), *Failure to Thrive and Malnutrition*,
https://doi.org/10.1007/978-3-031-14164-5_2

on how and what caregivers feed the child. A developmental evaluation may identify any developmental abnormalities associated with failure to thrive. Developmental delay may be an indicator of malnutrition, underlying neurological disorder, metabolic disorder, or psychosocial problem such as neglect that may contribute to or worsen failure to thrive [1].

Physical exam features seen in children with failure to thrive may include decreased subcutaneous fat in the face, arms, thighs, and buttocks as well as a decreased muscle mass. These areas will appear baggy or with wrinkles instead of healthy—full and curved. In severe cases of malnutrition, children may have dermatitis, hepatomegaly, cheilosis, or edema [2].

Lack of Calories: Not Enough In

In general, insufficient calories are the most common reason for failure to thrive [3]. A good dietary history is essential. Infants 0–8 months should receive approximately 100–115 calories/kg/day. Infants 8–12 months should receive approximately 85 calories/kg/day. The estimated daily nutritional need for toddlers is approximatedly 1000 calories per day based on Dietary Reference Intake/Sedentary guidelines [4].

Case 1

A 6-week-old infant male is brought to his primary care provider's office for concerns of poor weight gain. The patient is exclusively breast-fed. Mother states that the baby breastfeeds every 4 h for approximately 10 min. Mother states that the baby is already sleeping through the night. On exam, the patient is noted to have 10 g per day weight gain since birth. Physical exam notes normal vital signs. The weight is 3.8 kg and height is 55 cm. The WHO Z-score is −2. The patient has subcutaneous fat on the face, but little to no fat on the buttocks. The arms have small wrinkles along the triceps. Child is in no apparent distress and the remainder of the physical exam is normal.

The first step in evaluation is to determine if the patient is malnourished or not. This patient is moderately malnourished based on the weight for length Z-score of −2 as well as lack of subcutaneous fat on his face and buttocks. The next step is to determine the cause of his malnutrition. Is he having too little calories in, losing calories, or needs more calories/ has increased metabolic demand?

In a breastfeeding infant, insufficient milk intake may be due to insufficient milk production or inadequate milk transfer. Maternal factors or infant health conditions may prevent proper breast stimulation. A breastfeeding neonate should feed every 2–3 h or 8–12 times per day for 10–20 min each feed [5]. Direct observation of breastfeeding by a practitioner may help identify proper technique and production. If a large volume of milk is expressed after feeding, there may be concern for improper transfer of milk leading to decreased milk production by mother. If the infant is fussy or pulling away at breast, there may be concern for aversion possibly due to reflux or milk protein allergy.

Case Resolution Mother was referred to a lactation consultant and instructed to wake up the child at night for feeds. Infant was followed closely by providers and became more vigorous and started gaining weight.

Case 2

A 9-month old previously healthy male presents for checkup. Parents state he is doing well—taking 6–8 ounces of formula every 5 h and eating a jar of baby food three times a day. They are mixing the formula by adding 1 scoop of formula to 2 ounces of water. There are no problems with spitting up feeds. Parents state their child stools once a day and the stool is soft and brown. No developmental delays are noted on the exam and history. Past medical history is unremarkable. Baby was born term with no hospitalizations or chronic illnesses. Family history is unremarkable—patient lives at home with his parents and 1 older sibling. Vital signs are within normal limits except for a weight of 7.4 kg which plots to the fifth percentile. Physical exam findings are significant for a thin male with minimal subcutaneous fat. Growth curve is shown in Fig. 2.1.

Since the infant is formula fed, important questions to ask are the type of formula that is being used, how the formula is being mixed, and how many ounces are taken in 24 h. Ready-to-feed formulas generally have 19–20 kcal/30 mL (1 oz) and approximately 67–67 kcal/dL [2]. Asking about the maximum

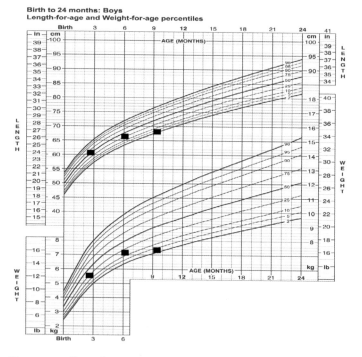

FIGURE 2.1 Growth curve

amount taken during a feed may help to evaluate if there is aversion. It is also important to ask who is feeding the baby and if there is any bottle propping which could lead to insufficient milk intake. Formula feeding should be ad lib. Usual weight gain is 25–30 g/day in the first 1–3 months of life. The rate of weight gain declines from 3 to 12 months of age [2, 4]. In general, weight growth velocity at 4–8 months 10–16 g/day and at 8–12 months average weight gain is 6–11 g/day [4].

Case Resolution Evaluation of the child's diet revealed that the patient was getting a total of 60 kcal/kg/day from a formula which was likely the result of his failure to thrive. Parents were given nutritional education/instructions and offered bottles more frequently and increased calories of baby foods. Child was followed and his weight improved on return visits with the provider.

Case 3

A 3-year-old female was referred to pediatric gastroenterology for no weight gain in 6 months. Her eating has decreased over the last year. She does not have diarrhea or vomiting, but she has been choking intermittently over the last year. She takes longer than usual to finish chewing her meals and she avoids eating bread or meats. She has been on a proton pump inhibitor for presumed reflux without any improvement in symptoms. Parents deny fevers or joint pain. She has eczema and one sibling has asthma.

The lack of weight gain in the case above was caused by a lack of calories taken in. Patients 2–6 years of age are expected to grow an average of 2–3 kg per year in weight and 5–8 cm in height per year [4]. Dysphagia and food impaction are common presenting symptoms of eosinophilic esophagitis (EoE). The child in the case manifested these symptoms by refusing to eat bread and meats: two foods that commonly are associated with dysphagia in EoE [6]. Upper endoscopy with biopsy is needed to make the appropriate diagnosis.

Case Resolution Because of choking in the setting of eczema with a family history of asthma, the gastroenterologist's suspicion of eosinophilic esophagitis (EoE) was high. An upper endoscopy confirmed the diagnosis. She was started on a course of oral swallowed budesonide and her weight has steadily increased over the last 2 months.

The most common presentation of EoE in toddlers is nausea/vomiting, dysphagia, abdominal pain, feeding disorders, heartburn, food impaction, and chest pain. The age of presentation varies from 6 months to 20 years. Eosinophilic esophagitis in children and adolescents have variable epidemiology, clinical presentation, and seasonal variation.

When a provider is concerned for decreased calories being consumed, they may ask the caregiver to record a 3-day food diary and consult a dietitian to calculate how many calories the child is eating. A toddler's birthweight usually triples by the first year of life and quadruples by the second year of life. Toddlers should consume three healthy meals and two snacks daily but may be easily distracted or self-limit their diet. WHO weight for length Z-scores can be used to determine the severity of malnutrition [7].

Failure to thrive is a multifactorial condition and food insecurity, caregiver depression, and child maltreatment should be considered in differential [8]. Up to 25% of reported cases of medical child abuse have presented as failure to thrive or anorexia. Several studies have shown the relationship between reported food allergies and medical child abuse due to extremely restrictive diets [9]. Table 2.1 Demonstrates questions providers may ask when lack of calories is on the differential for failure to thrive.

TABLE 2.1 Lack of calories

Lack of calories in differential	Questions or techniques that may help lead to diagnosis
Infant	
Improper mixing of formula	How is formula mixed?
Limiting volume of feeds	How many ounces? What is the feeding schedule? Does baby wake up at night to feed? How many ounces per feed?
Poor calorie formula	What is the baby getting for feeds? Anything other than commercial formula? Water? Juice?
Improper breastfeeding technique	Observe infant feed. A woman's breasts enlarge during pregnancy
Insufficient feeding due to aversion	Does the infant seem to pull away from the breast or bottle? Irritability after feeds? What is the maximum amount of feeds child will take per feed?
Insufficient Milk production	Failure to enlarge or minimal breast tissue on examination may clue the practitioner to a possible failure of lactation [5]
Neurologic disorder with impaired swallowing	Observe infant feed
Caregiver depression	Who is the primary caregiver? Are they waking up to feed child? Has the primary caregiver had postpartum depression screen?
Poverty	Any concerns for access to food? Is family stretching out formula because they cannot afford?
Child maltreatment	Who is primary caregiver? Any physical findings concerning of abuse? Severe food restrictions?

(continued)

TABLE 2.1 (continued)

Lack of calories in differential	Questions or techniques that may help lead to diagnosis
Toddler	
Juice consumption	How much juice does the child take per day?
Highly distractible child	Does the child sit down while eating? Is caregiver having to chase them around?
Dental caries	How often does the patient have teeth brushed? Do they seem to favor soft foods? Any pain while eating? Any foul odor in breath?
Poor diet/severe food restrictions	Ask for detailed dietary history. Any food allergies? Any food modifications?

Too Many Calories Out

Case 4

A 3-month-old female has been referred to the pediatric gastroenterologist for malnutrition. She is formula fed. The formula is a soy formula. She takes in an average of 5 ounces per feed by mouth every 3–4 h for a total of 6 feeds a day. This is an average of 30 ounces per day and a total of 600 calories per day (150 kcal/kg/day). Parents describe moderate volume emesis that occurs immediately after feeds. She weighs 4 kg and her height is 57 cm; Z-score is −3 [10].

In the case above failure to thrive may be due to persistent vomiting or malabsorptive states. The approach to an infant with vomiting begins with asking a few key questions. History should include age of onset, feeding and dietary history (volume of feed, length of feed, breastfeeding or type of formula and how it is mixed, additives, timing of feeds and any restrictions due to food allergies?), pattern of regurgitation/vomiting (does it occur immediately after feeds or long after meals or only at night?), and consistency of emesis (digested vs.

undigested, bilious, bloody?). Environmental factors also play a role in vomiting, including family medical history and environmental triggers such as family/social stressors. Physiologic gastroesophageal reflux (GER) typically starts between 1 week and 6 months of age. Any vomiting symptoms after 6 months of age or persisting/worsening after 12–18 months should be investigated. Concerning symptoms include weight loss, irritability/pain, as well as accompanying neurological symptoms such as budging fontanelle, increasing head circumference, seizures, and macro/microcephaly. Morning vomiting may suggest increased intracranial pressure and bilious vomiting is concerning for intestinal obstruction. Associated diarrhea may suggest a food protein-induced enteropathy [11]. Diarrhea is not necessary to make the diagnosis of milk protein enteropathy.

Case Resolution Given a history of vomiting immediately after feeds, pyloric stenosis was high on differential. Patient had ultrasound which revealed pyloric stenosis. Patient had pyloromyotomy and symptoms resolved.

Case 5

A 5-month-old term male was diagnosed with colic by his pediatrician. He presents to pediatric gastroenterology clinic for poor weight gain. He is exclusively breastfed and has been irritable during breastfeeding over the last 3 months. During this time, his spitting up has worsened as he spits up with each feed and arches his back after each episode. He pushes away the breast during feeds. He stools nearly with each feed. Parents describe stools as non-bloody, loose, and intermittently mucoid.

Additional history reveals a family history significant for brother with asthma and mother with eczema. Social history is unremarkable. Child weighs 5 kg, length is 61 cm, and weight-for-length Z-score is −2.82. His FOC and vitals are normal. Physical exam is remarkable for child's arms and buttocks not being full but instead wrinkled. Otherwise physical exam is unremarkable.

Diarrhea may be a result of malabsorption of three main nutrients: carbohydrates, protein, or fat. When asking about history of diarrhea it is important to ask about frequency and consistency (mucous, color, blood). This patient is spitting up and having loose stools, which represent a loss of calories (too many calories going out). The child's exam, with the exception of lack of subcutaneous fat, was unremarkable making the case for an increase in metabolic demand less likely. Given this infant's irritability and arching with feeding, he has reflux with associated Sandifer syndrome; the loose, mucoid stool points us less toward colic and more in the direction of milk protein enteropathy or allergic colitis. This patient may also have a component of decreased calories as he pushes away the breast during feeding and his ideal caloric intake is not likely being met.

Allergic colitis typically refers to non-IgE-mediated food allergy and encompasses a wide range of disorders affecting the gastrointestinal tract including food protein-induced enterocolitis syndrome (FPIES), food protein-induced allergic proctocolitis (FPIAP), food protein-induced enteropathy (FPE), and celiac disease. Typically, symptoms present in the first 3–6 months of life [12]. FPIES to solid foods usually starts at 4–7 months and typically present when chronic symptoms develop in young infants with regular intake of food (such as infant formula) and include intermittent but progressive emesis, diarrhea (with or without blood), and failure to thrive [12]. The most common food allergen in this condition is cow's milk or soy.

Case Resolution Diagnosis of milk protein-induced enteropathy was made. The patient's mother saw a registered dietitian to discuss avoidance of dairy and soy. On follow-up visit with pediatrician, mother notes child is eating well and comfortable during feeds with elimination of soy and dairy. He no longer spits up and stools once every other day; bowel movements are soft and without mucus. The patient was seen 1 and 2 months later with normalization of his weight and normal weight for length Z-score.

TABLE 2.2 Too many calories out

Vomiting: too many calories out

Vomiting	Questions that may lead to diagnosis
Gastroesophageal reflux disease	Vomiting after feeds, arching of back (Sandifer syndrome), fussiness
Pyloric stenosis	Projectile vomiting? Symptoms younger than 3 months of age, vomiting with feeds or after feeds, infant hungry after vomiting, dehydration, belching, family history of pyloric stenosis
Neurologic: Increased intracranial pressure	History of trauma? Vomiting in morning? Bulging Fontanelle?
Vascular ring	Vomiting during feeds or immediately after feeds. Low volume of feeds per meal
Infectious	Duration?

The allergy in a child with milk protein allergy may be an allergy to cow's milk, soy milk, hydrolyzed casein protein and maternal dietary proteins. It may take 2–4 weeks for the protein to clear the mother's milk supply however symptoms can improve within 48–72 h [13]. If the mother starts the restricted diet and continues to breastfeed, the child is expected to remain symptomatic during the course of diet elimination. There should be an improvement in temperament, frequency of stool, and consistency stool as the enteric inflammation improves. Table 2.2 is a tool that providers may use if concerns that patient is losing too many calories resulting in failure to thrive.

Diarrhea: too many calories out

Diarrhea	Questions that may lead to diagnosis
Infectious • Bacterial • Viral • Parasitic • Bacterial overgrowth	Duration? Sick contacts? History of surgeries? Any stool studies?

Diarrhea: too many calories out	
Diarrhea	**Questions that may lead to diagnosis**
Noninfectious: malabsorptive states	

• Protein malabsorption
  – Food protein-induced enterocolitis syndrome (FPIES)
  – Food protein-induced allergic proctocolitis (FPIAP)
  – Food protein-induced enteropathy (FPE)
	Mucous and/or blood in stool? Irritability after feeds? Oral aversion during feeds? Eczema? Family history of asthma and/or eczema?

• Fat Malabsorption – Pancreatic insufficiency	History of frequent pancreatitis? Pancreatic abnormality

• Carbohydrate malabsorption
  – Celiac disease
  – High osmotic load
	Diarrhea starts at time of solid food introduction? Juice intake?

• Inflammatory bowel disease	Bloody stools? Mucoid stools? Fever? Joint pain? Chronic course of weight loss? Stunting in height? Anemia?
• Motility disorder – Hirschsprung	Passed stool in the first 24–48 h of life? Fever? Abdominal distention?

Case 6

A 2 1/2-year-old female was referred to pediatric gastroenterology for chronic constipation, abdominal pain, and lack of weight gain. Patient stools once every 3 days; the stools are hard and not associated with blood. Constipation is associated with abdominal distention that worsens as the day progresses. The distention does not resolve completely after passing stool. Child is 15th percentile for weight and height. Her weight for length Z-score is normal, but she has not gained weight in 6 months; her height has also not increased. Her past medical history and social history are unremarkable. Family medical history is significant for mother with hypothyroidism and maternal uncle who is the "thinnest in the family" and "has a lot of gas." Vital signs are normal. Physical examination is remarkable for abdominal distention that is tympanic and palpable stools.

Constipation is a common problem in pediatrics. A red flag for diagnoses beyond constipation is when malnutrition is a part of the clinical picture. Abdominal distention is also common in constipation; however, the distention should improve after stooling. In this case, the distention was progressive throughout the day and was associated with abdominal pain.

Case Resolution Laboratory workup revealed a normal electrolyte and complete blood count. Thyroid studies were normal. A normal total IgA and elevated titers of tissue transglutaminase (IgA tTG) of 12 IU/mL led the gastroenterologist to schedule an esophagogastroduodenoscopy (EGD); EGD biopsy confirmed diagnosis of celiac disease. The patient's uncle was later also found to have celiac disease. After dietary therapy, constipation management, and confirmation of celiac disease, the patient had catch up growth and abdominal distention resolved.

The differential for chronic constipation is large and history/physical exam is key in identifying potential underlying causes. Evaluation of electrolytes, metabolic causes of hypomotility (hypothyroid), and causes of inflammation should be taken into consideration when evaluating chronic constipation.

Increased Metabolic Demand

Case 7

A 4-month-old female patient with Down Syndrome was referred to a pediatric gastroenterologist for malnutrition. She has grown an average of 15 g/day over the last 1 month. She is formula fed and is consuming an average of 110 calories/kg/day. She is not fussy, does not vomit, and does not have diarrhea. Her stools are soft and seedy without mucus. She is below 3% on the Down Syndrome growth chart and she is less than 3% on height. She has normal vitals however physical exam reveals a mid-systolic murmur with wide and fixed splitting of second heart sound consistent with Atrial Septal Defect (ASD).

When children exhibit persistent failure to thrive after insufficient calorie intake is ruled out and there is no concern for losing excessive calories, the next step is to consider increased metabolic demand. The child in case above most likely has an increase in caloric demand from an ASD.

Case Resolution   Child was found to have a large ASD. Patient's caloric intake was increased to 150 kcal/kg/day with concentrated feeds and child began to gain weight. Patient was followed closely by Gastroenterology and Cardiology to make sure there was no volume overload and her weight improved over time.

Increased metabolic demand may be due to cardiac, pulmonary, renal, neurologic disease, or inborn errors of metabolism. Family history is important when considering the differential of malabsorption or metabolic disorder contributing to failure to thrive. Reviewing the newborn screen is helpful for assessing genetic or metabolic disorders when reviewing history, however, screening does not have 100% sensitivity or specificity and the number of metabolic disorders screened varies from one state to another [8, 14].

Case 8

A 6-month-old male is admitted to the hospital for lethargy and seizures. He was born term. On day 3 of life, child had vomiting with high anion gap metabolic acidosis and was treated as sepsis. After being discharged 2 weeks later from the NICU, patient continued to have vomiting and poor weight gain. Patient did not respond to reflux medications. He developed seizures at 4 months of age and was noted to have a high anion gap acidosis and ketonuria. Physical exam showed lethargy, axial hypotonia, and movement disorder.

Inborn errors of metabolism should be considered in infants who present with sepsis-like pictures after looking well the first 24–48 h of life. Some may present later when dietary changes add more protein to the diet or during period of catabolism, such as when the infant is sick or starts sleeping through the night. Patients may also present with developmental delay or regression. Physical exam may reveal organomegaly or mild dysmorphic or coarse facial features [14]. Family history of siblings with similar illnesses or deaths from unidentified pathogen sepsis may also be identified. History of consanguinity can increase risk of autosomal recessive disorders.

All 50 states including the District of Columbia screen for cystic fibrosis (CF), however, several factors may lead to missing a diagnosis of CF in the early newborn period. Examples may be not obtaining newborn screen (such as home birth), insufficient sample, or lab error. In addition, the number of CF mutations on the screening panel varies from state to state [15].

Case Resolution Due to high anion gap, physical exam findings, and seizures, the case above is highly suggestive of a metabolic disorder. Patient was worked up by genetics and results of plasma amino acid, urine organic acid, and plasma acylcarnitine revealed diagnosis of propionic academia [14].

Table 2.3 demonstrates questions providers may ask if there is concerned for increased demand in differential for failure to thrive.

In summary, failure to thrive is multifactorial. Most common is not enough calories, however, using the systemic approach of calories in, calories out, or increased caloric demand can help the clinician come to the diagnosis (Table 2.4) [16].

TABLE 2.3 Increased demand for diagnosis

Increased demand	Questions that may lead to diagnosis
Cardiac	Eating expected amounts? Fatigue during eating? Cyanosis? Sweating during feeds?
Pulmonary Cystic fibrosis	Foul smelling stools, diarrhea, frequent infections, recurrent pneumonias
Chronic infections	Concern for immunodeficiency? Family history of immune deficiency, chronic diarrhea, persistent thrush, concern for HIV, recurrent pneumonias, opportunistic infections
Inborn error of metabolism	Dysmorphic facial features? Seizures? History of consanguinity? Developmental delay? High anion gap acidosis, lactic acidosis, hypoketotic hypoglycemia

TABLE 2.4 Differential diagnosis of failure to thrive summary

Diagnosis	Clinical features	Initial laboratory tests and evaluations
Inadequate calorie intake		
Cleft palate	Milk regurgitation through nose HEENT examination	Speech/swallow consult
Excess juice consumption	Dietary history	None
Incorrect formula preparation	Dietary history History of economic pressures	CBC, electrolytes
Oromotor dysfunction	Observation of feedings	Speech/swallow consult
Poor feeding technique	Observation of feeding	Observe patient feeding
Psychosocial— Insufficient food	Stressors in home	CBC, electrolytes Social work consult
Inadequate caloric absorption/utilization		
Celiac disease	Family historyDiarrhea	CBC, albumin Anti-tissue transglutaminase (anti-TTG) Stool pH, reducing substances, fecal fats
Cystic fibrosis	Family history Abnormal newborn screen Respiratory symptoms Diarrhea	Review newborn screen Sweat test Stool pH, reducing substances and fecal fats

(continued)

TABLE 2.4 (continued)

Diagnosis	Clinical features	Initial laboratory tests and evaluations
Gastroesophageal reflux	Vomiting history	Response to treatment ± swallowing study or pH probe
Increased intracranial pressure	Vomiting history Cushing triad Abnormal neurologic exam	Head CT Neurology consult
Inflammatory bowel disease	Family history Diarrhea, bloody stools	CBC, ESR/CRP, albumin Stool occult blood
Liver disease	Jaundice Diarrhea	Liver function tests Hepatitis serologies
Milk protein allergy/ enteropathy	Family history Vomiting history Diarrhea, bloody stools Eczema	Stool occult blood GI consult Possible endoscopy
Increased calorie requirements		
Adrenal diseases	Vomiting, diarrhea Hyperpigmentation Hypotension	Chemistry Glucose
Blood disorders	Fatigue Pallor	CBC
Cardiopulmonary diseases	Fatigue, especially with feeds Respiratory illnesses	Chest X-ray EKG and echocardiogram
Diabetes mellitus	Polydipsia, polyuria, polyphagia	Chemistry, fasting glucose Urinalysis

TABLE 2.4 (continued)

Diagnosis	Clinical features	Initial laboratory tests and evaluations
Genetic diseases	Family history Dysmorphic features	Specific for suspected disease
Hyperthyroidism	Fatigue, increased sweating, polyphagia Nervousness, sleep disturbance Diarrhea, tachycardia, exophthalmos	Thyroid studies
Renal tubular acidosis	Normal anion gap metabolic acidosis	Venous blood gas and urinalysis (compare serum and urine pH)

As described in Vachani, V. Failure to Thrive: Caring for the Hospitalized Child: A Handbook of Inpatient Pediatrics, Editors Gershel and Rauch. 2013, 485–491

References

1. Homan GJ. Failure to thrive: a practical guide. Am Fam Physician. 2016;94(4):295–9.
2. Kleigman R. In: Fortin K, Downes A, editors. Nelson textbook of pediatrics. 21st ed. Philadelphia, PA: Elsevier; 2020.
3. Larson-Nath CM, Goday PS. Failure to thrive: a prospective study in a pediatric gastroenterology clinic. J Pediatr Gastroenterol Nutr. 2016;62(6):907–13.
4. Texas Children's Hospital. In: Mills J, Ramsey E, Rich S, Trout S, Bunting KD, editors. Texas children's hospital pediatric nutrition guide. 12th ed. Houston, TX: Texas Children's Hospital; 2019.
5. Gabbe SM. Obstetrics: normal and problem pregnancies. In: Newton ER, editor. Lactation and breastfeeding. 7th ed. Philadelphia, PA: Elsevier; 2017. p. 517–48.
6. Straumann A, Aceves SS, Blanchard C, Collins MH, Furuta GT, Hirano I, et al. Pediatric and adult eosinophilic esophagitis: similarities and differences. Allergy. 2012;67(4):477–90.

7. WHO. Child growth standards and the identification of severe acute malnutrition in infants and children: a joint statement by the World Health Organization and the United Nations Children's Fund. Geneva: World Health Organization; 2009.

8. Jaffe AC. Failure to thrive: current clinical concepts. Pediatr Rev. 2011;32(3):100–8.

9. Mash C, Frazier T, Nowacki A, Worley S, Goldfarb J. Development of a risk-stratification tool for medical child abuse in failure to thrive. Pediatrics. 2011;128(6):e1467–e73.

10. Kleinman R, Goulet O-J, Mieli-Viergani G, Sanderson M, Ian Sherman P, Schneider B. Walker's pediatric gastrointestinal disease. 6th ed. Raleigh, NC: People's Medical Publishing House; 2018.

11. Rosen R, Vandenplas Y, Singendonk M, Cabana M, DiLorenzo C, Gottrand F, et al. Pediatric gastroesophageal reflux clinical practice guidelines: joint recommendations of the North American Society for Pediatric Gastroenterology, Hepatology, and Nutrition and the European Society for Pediatric Gastroenterology, Hepatology, and Nutrition. J Pediatr Gastroenterol Nutr. 2018;66(3):516–54.

12. Nowak-Węgrzyn A, Katz Y, Mehr SS, Koletzko S. Non-IgE-mediated gastrointestinal food allergy. J Allergy Clin Immunol. 2015;135(5):1114–24.

13. Lake AM. Dietary protein enterocolitis. Immunol Allergy Clin N Am. 1999;19:553–61.

14. Ficicioglu C, An Haack K. Failure to thrive: when to suspect inborn errors of metabolism. Pediatrics. 2009;124(3):972–9.

15. Rock MJ, Levy H, Zaleski C, Farrell PM. Factors accounting for a missed diagnosis of cystic fibrosis after newborn screening. Pediatr Pulmonol. 2011;46(12):1166–74.

16. Vachani V. Failure to thrive: caring for the hospitalized child. In: Gershel C, Rauch DA, editors. A handbook of inpatient pediatrics. American Academy of Pediatrics; 2013. p. 485–91.

Chapter 3
Growth Assessment and Its Significance

Bridget Dowd Kiernan and Maria Mascarenhas

Growth assessment—the interpretation of anthropometric growth measurements including length/height, weight, head circumference, weight-for-length, and body mass index—is an important part of nutritional assessment and a critical component of clinical care for all pediatric patients. Assessment of anthropometric measures is a noninvasive, safe, and inexpensive tool that allows for efficient screening for malnutrition in children [1]. While there is no single direct measure of nutrition, growth is a sign of health and nutritional status. Growth velocity acceleration or deceleration, when out of the range of normal, can be a harbinger of malnutrition at times secondary to various disease states. Growth in utero and postnatally from the neonatal period through infancy, childhood, adolescence, and young adulthood is vitally important for the promotion of health and human development. The most important measurements needed for growth assessment are (1) recumbent length or height, (2) weight, and (3) head circumference. These fundamental anthropometric measures should be obtained and interpreted at each well child visit,

B. D. Kiernan (✉) · M. Mascarenhas
Division of Gastroenterology, Hassenfeld Children's Hospital at NYU Langone Health, New York, NY, USA
e-mail: Bridget.Kiernan@nyulangone.org;
MASCARENHAS@email.chop.edu

J. G. Vachani (ed.), *Failure to Thrive and Malnutrition*,
https://doi.org/10.1007/978-3-031-14164-5_3

and are typically sufficient for growth assessment. Additional anthropometric measurements are helpful in many specific situations. Table 3.1 lists the main components of growth assessment.

TABLE 3.1 Components of growth assessment

Anthropometric indicator	Equipment/comments
Weight	Calibrated weighing scale; report to 1 g (0.001 kg) in infants, 0.01 kg in children/adolescents
Length/height	Report to 0.1 cm ≤24 months: Length via infantometer, plot on WHO curve [2] >24 months: Height via stadiometer, plot on CDC curve [3]
Head circumference	Tape measure; report widest measurement to 0.1 cm <24–36 months: Plot on WHO [2] >24–36 months until 18 years: Plot on CDC [3] >18 years: Plot on Nellhaus [4]
Weight-for-length	0–36 months: Plot on WHO curve [2]
Body mass index (BMI)	BMI = Weight in kg/(height in m)^2: Plot on CDC [3]
Mid-parental target height	Girls: [(Father's height − 13) + Mother's height]/2 Boys: [(Mother's height + 13) + Father's height]/2 (±2 SDs around target height is ±8.5 cm or 3.35 in.) [5]
Growth velocity	Weight velocity curve [6, 7]
	Height velocity curve [8]
Bone age	Assessment of growth based on stage of skeletal bone development compared to references for age [9–12]

Obtaining Measurements

Measurement accuracy and reliability are extremely important as the data obtained influences management. All anthropometric devices need to be inspected and calibrated regularly based on standards to prevent variation or errors in measurements secondary to wear and tear of equipment. Even tape measures require replacement when no longer meeting standards. Stadiometers and electronic weight scales require regular calibration with a calibration bar and weights, respectively. Medical assistants, nurses, and other health care professionals who perform and report these measurements require training in technique and consistency to achieve reproducible measurements. At times, in an uncooperative patient, two persons and adequate time are necessary to perform measurements correctly. Recumbent length and height measurements vary, and length measurements are typically slightly larger than height measurements in the same patient. It is important to plot length and height on the appropriate growth chart as discussed later in this chapter.

Weight

Infants should be undressed entirely and weighed in the nude without a diaper on. Report infants' weight to the nearest gram (1 g = 0.001 kg). Older children may wear light clothing with bare feet after taking their shoes off. Report children's weight to the nearest 0.1 kg. Ideally, longitudinal measurements are obtained on the same scale under similar circumstances such as time of day. Measurements at home may vary from those taken at a pediatrician or subspecialist's office. Interpret measurements from each scale with caution and compare them to previous measurements on that same scale. Wheelchair accessible scales allow measurement with and without the child in the wheelchair to determine the child's weight. Note the weight of the wheelchair in the patient's chart and whether there is any additional equipment attached to the chair.

Length/Height

To measure stature, a patient's appropriate position is with the head in the Frankfort plane. The Frankfort plane includes the line from the lower border of the orbit to the auditory meatus. This should be perpendicular to ground or parallel to the headboard when using a stadiometer to measure height, and perpendicular to the backboard when using an infantometer to measure recumbent length. Infants and children up until 2 years old, or those who cannot stand, should have recumbent length measured lying down with their head against the headboard and their legs stretched outward with knees flat and feet at a 90° angle from the backboard, parallel to the footboard.

Once a child is 2 years or older and can stand steadily and distribute their weight evenly, their height measurement should be performed standing using a stadiometer. The back of the head, shoulders, buttocks, and heels are all placed against the stadiometer, with bare feet flat on the floor. The knees also need to be touched and the legs must be straight. The head position still needs to be in the Frankfort plane, as discussed above, because moving the head or neck slightly out of this plane will distort the measurement. Similarly, any hairpieces or head ornaments on top of their heads need to be removed. Report stature to the nearest 0.1 cm.

Head Circumference

To obtain head circumference, secure a tape measure above the supraorbital ridge with one hand and then wrap it around the head with the other hand ensuring that it is even and flat around the back of the skull. Adjust the position of the tape measure until the largest circumference measurement of the head is found, and report it to the nearest 0.1 cm. Head circumference should be measured until 36 months of age in all children, and beyond for certain patients as necessary per the American Academy of Pediatrics (AAP), World Health

Organization (WHO), and Centers for Disease Control (CDC) recommendations [1, 3, 13]. Patients with microcephaly or macrocephaly should have head circumference measured beyond 3 years of age to monitor for changes. WHO and CDC head circumference normative values go up to 36 months of age; Nellhaus charts exist for older children and are available in some electronic health records [4].

Alternative Height Measures

When linear length/height cannot be measured in children who are unable to stand or lay flat—for example, due to severe contractures, scoliosis, or skeletal abnormalities—alternative segmental measures of the extremities or trunk can be used to estimate stature [14]. These include sitting height, arm span, ulnar length, upper arm length, knee height, and tibial length. See Table 3.2 for details. Measure sitting height with the patient's arms relaxed at the patient's sides while seated on a box set up against the stadiometer. The distance from the top of the head to the top of the sitting surface (box) represents sitting height. Children less than 6 years of age who are unable to stand, can lay flat, and do not have cerebral palsy (CP) or neurologic impairment (NI) should have recumbent length measured on an infantometer or length board. Arm span is used to calculate estimated stature in children who do not have CP/NI and cannot lay flat, but can spread their arms laterally to each side [15]. In patients with CP or NI, the preferred alternate height measure is knee height [17]. This can also be used for children without CP/NI [18]. Knee height is measured from the top of the thigh to the bottom of a foot placed flat on the floor [19]. In children with CP/NI and abnormal skeletal anatomy or contractures of the lower extremities who cannot place their feet flat on the ground, tibial length is helpful. Tibial length is the distance between the tibial tubercle and the medial malleolus with the leg in any position [20, 21].

TABLE 3.2 Measures for estimation of stature and body composition

Stature

Measurement	Age (years)	Equations for estimation of predicted stature, S (cm)
Recumbent Length [14]	0–6	Infantometer or length board on a flat surface, to 0.1 cm
Arm span (AS) [15, 16]	>6	Female: $[0.619 \times AS] + [1.593 \times age] + 36.976 = S$ Male: $[0.829 \times AS] + [0.721 \times age] + 16.258 = S$
Knee height (KH) [14, 17–19]	0–12 with CP/NI[a]	$[2.69 \times KH] + 24.2 = S$
	12–18 with CP/NI, 6–18 typically developing [19]	African American girl: $[2.02 \times KH] + 46.59 = S$ African American boy: $[2.18 \times KH] + 39.60 = S$ Caucasian girl: $[2.15 \times KH] + 43.21 = S$ Caucasian boy: $[2.22 \times KH] + 40.54 = S$
	19–60 [19]	African American woman: $[1.86 \times KH] - [0.06 \times age] + 68.10 = S$ Caucasian woman: $[1.87 \times KH] - [0.06 \times age] + 70.25 = S$ African American man: $[1.79 \times KH] + 73.42 = S$ Caucasian man: $[1.88 \times KH] + 71.85 = S$

TABLE 3.2 (continued)

Tibial length (TL) [14, 16, 20, 21]	0–12 with CP/NI	Girl: $[2.771 \times TL] + [1.457 \times age] + 37.748 = S$ Boy: $[2.758 \times TL] + [1.717 \times age] + 36.509 = S$
	All	Female: $[2.691 \times TL] + 65.344 = S$ Male: $[2.575 \times TL] + 71.361 = S$
Leg Length [18]	All	Female: $[2.473 \times leg\ length] + [1.187 \times age] + 21.151 = S$ Male: $[2.423 \times leg\ length] + [1.327 \times age] + 21.818 = S$
Ulnar length (U) [16]	5–19 typically developing [16]	Girl: $[4.459 \times U] + [1.315 \times age] + 31.485 = S$ Boy: $[4.605 \times U] + [1.308 \times age] + 28.003 = S$
Forearm Length [18]	All	Female: $[2.908 \times forearm\ length] + [1.147 \times age] + 21.167 = S$ Male: $[2.904 \times forearm\ length] + [1.193 \times age] + 20.432 = S$
Upper arm length (UAL) [14]	0–12 with CP/NI	$[4.35 \times UAL] + 21.8 = S$
	All	Female: $[2.908 \times UAL] + [1.147 \times age] + 21.167 = S$ Male: $[2.904 \times UAL] + [1.193 \times age] + 20.432 = S$
Sitting height (SH) [22]	All	Crown rump length in sitting position

(continued)

TABLE 3.2 (continued)

Body composition

Measurement		Equations
Arm Anthropometry [23–25]	Mid-upper arm circumference (MAC) [24]	Arm area, AA (mm²) = $$\frac{\pi}{4} \times \left[\frac{MAC}{\pi}\right]^2$$ Arm muscle area, AMA (mm²) = $\dfrac{(MAC - \pi T)^2}{4\pi}$ Arm fat area, AFA (mm²) = AA − AMA [25]
		Triceps skinfold thickness (TSFT) [26]
Dual-energy X-ray absorptiometry (DXA)		Total body less head scan allows calculation of percent body fat by measuring bone mass and tissue mass, which is subdivided into fat-free non-skeletal mass and fat mass [27, 28]
Waist circumference		Indicates risk of insulin resistance [1]

[a]P/NI: CP = cerebral palsy, NI = neurologic impairment. Patients without CP/N: 0–6 years, obtain recumbent length measured lying down if they can lay flat; >6 years, preferred measurement is arm span (AS), followed by knee height (KH). Patients with CP/NI at any age: KH is the preferred measurement, followed by tibial length (TL) for those 0–12 years old

Patients for whom neither length nor lower extremity measurements are appropriate due to neuromuscular weakness, or lower extremity joint or spinal deformities, upper extremity measurements are useful. Upper extremities may be less severely impacted than lower extremities by high spinal lesions. In those 6–18 years old, ulnar length is useful [16]. Ulnar length is determined with an anthropometer or a steel, plastic, or paper tape measure. Published equations allow estimation of stature using an alternate measure to length or recumbent height such as ulnar length, arm span, knee height or tibial length. The equations provide estimate of stature that can be assessed by comparing to growth curves [16]. See Table 3.2 for equations with these various segmental measures.

Bone Age

There are two major methods for bone age assessment; the first was described by Greulich and Pyle [9], and the other by Tanner and Whitehouse, most recently updated in the Tanner–Whitehouse 3 (TW3) method [9–12]. Bone age is reported in years and months based on radiographic images of a child's ossification centers in the left hand (including the wrist and fingers). The bone age is the age at which the bones of normally developing children exhibit the stage of ossification seen in the patient's left-hand X-ray. Interpretation involves comparing the bone age along with standard deviations with the patient's chronological age and sexual maturity. Bone age that falls outside of 2 standard deviations away from the normal range for their age is abnormal. Bone maturation assessment at one moment in time or over time may allow estimation of predicted ultimate height potential or identification of a potential window or lack thereof for catch-up growth prior to closure of growth plates [12]. Other measures of body and bone composition are also helpful, several of which are discussed below.

Body Composition

Upper Arm Anthropometry

Upper arm anthropometry is a particularly valuable anthropometric tool to assess risk for malnutrition and monitor nutritional status. It is very useful in multiple scenarios including hospitalized or critically ill patients, in resource-limited settings, in times of crisis, or in patients with edema or anasarca. Since fluid overload prevents proper interpretation of weight measurements, the upper arm is the best site for anthropometric measures of nutritional status in these patients as the lower extremities tend to have more dependent edema from gravity. Arm measurements are also helpful when linear growth measurements are not available. When stadiometers or scales are not available, or their use is precluded by clinical circumstances, arm anthropometry is an effective and efficient way to screen children for malnutrition with only a tape measure and/or calipers, which are portable. This is especially helpful in resource-limited settings as head circumference and mid-upper arm circumference (MUAC or MAC) can both be measured with just a measuring tape.

Arm anthropometry is most often performed by registered dietitians/nutritionists trained in proper techniques. MUAC is the circumference of the upper arm, measured at the mid-point between the tip of the elbow (olecranon), and the tip of the shoulder (acromion), with the elbow relaxed and the arm hanging freely [23, 29–32]. A tape measure wrapped around the arm on the skin surface without compressing the skin measures the circumference. Report MUAC to the nearest 0.1 cm [24, 33].

In the same location as MUAC on the mid-upper arm, at the posterior aspect over the triceps muscle, triceps skinfold thickness (TSFT) is measured with Holtain calipers with the patient standing upright with the arm dangling and relaxed [25, 26]. Skin and subcutaneous tissue thickness are measured on the right side of the body for consistency. In addition to the upper arm, other locations on the right side of the body can also be used, such as subscapular skinfold thickness (SSFT). Use SSFT in addition to TSFT to aid interpretation of subcutaneous fat stores. Report skinfolds to the nearest 0.1 mm.

Upper arm muscle mass area (AMA) and fat stores (AFA) are calculated from MUAC and TSFT, and compared to reference data for age [24]. MUAC and TSF are plotted by age on National Center for Health Statistics (NCHS) curves made from normative reference data, which allows assessment of nutrient stores based on body composition [24, 26].

MUAC and skinfold thicknesses are indicators of nutritional status and body composition since they allow estimation of skeletal muscle mass and subcutaneous fat stores [33].

These should be followed over time for valuable adjunctive anthropometric assessments in addition to routine evaluation and monitoring of patients at risk for malnutrition.

Bone Densitometry

Dual-energy X-ray absorptiometry (DXA scan) can be used to measure body composition. Scans of the body allow estimation of percent body fat by calculating the bone mass and soft-tissue mass, as well as its proportion of fat-free lean muscle mass. This can be performed in children 3 years of age and older as an indication of body composition [34, 35].

Body Mass Index

Body mass index (BMI) is weight in kilograms divided by the height in meters, squared. In children, BMI percentiles and Z-scores are used from 2 to 20 years of age, with BMI-for-age percentile between 5th and 85th classified as normal, 85th and 95th as overweight, greater than 95th as obese, and less than fifth as underweight. In adults (>20 years of age), the actual BMI number is used with cutoff values for BMI categories (underweight, normal weight, overweight, obese, and morbidly obese). BMI < 18.5 in adults represents underweight, BMI between 18.5 and 24.9 normal, BMI between 25 and 29.9 overweight and >30 obese. See Table 3.3.

Waist Circumference

Waist circumference is measured by measuring the body circumference below the ribs. Waist circumference above reference ranges has been shown to correlate with risk of insulin resistance and metabolic syndrome [1].

Table 3.3 Pediatric BMI classification

BMI-for-age	Recommended terminology
<5th percentile	Underweight
5th to <85th percentile	Healthy weight
85th to <95th percentile	Overweight
≥ 95th percentile to <120% of 95th percentile	Obesity class 1
≥ 120% to <140% of 95th percentile or adult BMI 35 to <40 kg/m^2	Severe obesity class 2 [36]
≥ 140% of the 95th percentile or adult BMI ≥ 40.0 kg/m^2	Severe obesity class 3 [36]

Frequency of Monitoring

From birth to 36 months of age, measurement of length, weight, and head circumference is part of every well child visit. After that, length/height and weight are measured at every well visit, with head circumference only if indicated.

Hospitalized patients need more frequent growth monitoring than outpatients. Patients on parenteral nutrition (PN) also need more frequent assessment of their weights. See Table 3.4 for a summary of recommended growth assessment frequency for outpatients per the AAP recommendations for preventive pediatric health care and for inpatients based on our local practice [1].

Table 3.4 Anthropometric measurement frequency recommendations. (Additional measurements may be necessary if circumstances suggest variations from normal. This is based on the 2016 Recommendations for Preventive Pediatric Health Care, American Academy of Pediatrics)

Outpatient well child [1]			
Age	Weight	Length/height	Head circumference
Infants from birth to 2 months	At 3–5 days of age and again by 1 month, then once per month	At 3–5 days of age and again by 1 month, then once per month	At 3–5 days of age and by 1 month, then once per month
2–6 months	Every 2 months	Every 2 months	Every 2 months
6–24 months	Every 3 months	Every 3 months	Every 3 months
2–6 years	Every year	Every year	As indicated
6–10 years	Every 1–2 years	Every 1–2 years	As indicated
>11 years	Every year	Every year	As indicated

(continued)

TABLE 3.4 (continued)

Inpatient

Age	Weight		Length/height	Head circumference
	Not on parenteral nutrition	On parenteral nutrition		
Preterm infant	Daily or as ordered	Daily	Weekly	Weekly
Term infant to 12 months	2 times per week	Daily	Monthly	Monthly
12–24 months	Weekly	2 times per week	Monthly	Monthly
2–20 years	Weekly	2 times per week	Monthly	As indicated
Adults >20 years	Weekly	2 times per week	On admission	As indicated

Table adapted from the CHOP Clinical Pathway for Inpatient Pediatric Malnutrition [37]. https://www.chop.edu/clinical-pathway/malnutrition-undernutrition-monitor-anthropometrics#

Growth Charts

There are genetic and cultural growth differences seen in different ethnic and geographic populations and therefore it is important that growth charts reflect the populations for which they are used. Growth assessment of each patient requires the use of the appropriate growth charts for an individual's most representative population. In the United States (U.S.), WHO charts are used as a growth standard for infants up until 2 years of age, and CDC growth charts are used for growth assessment from 2 to 20 years of age.

NCHS growth charts developed in the late 1970s were based on a longitudinal sample of children with European ancestry from one community in the United States from birth to 3 years, so they were not reflective of diverse populations of American children. Subsequently, CDC published growth charts in 2000 that are more representative of multi-ethnic US populations. The descriptive charts are based on large samples of cross-sectional data from 0 to 20 year old between 1970s and early 1990s from the whole country comprised of 74% non-Hispanic whites, 14% non-Hispanic blacks, 9% Hispanics, 2% Asian, and 1% Native American. Low birth weight (LBW) infants (less than 2500 g at birth), were included, but not very low birth weight (VLBW) infants (less than 1500 g at birth). These children were both formula and breastfed (one-third were breastfed for 3 months). CDC growth charts include 3rd and 97th percentiles, and curves for BMI.

In 2010, the WHO Multicenter Growth Reference Study (MGRS) published prescriptive growth charts including height velocity based on an international longitudinal sample of 8500 healthy mostly breastfed infants (including LBW, excluding multiples) through 5 years old living in optimal environmental conditions from 1997 to 2003. Most infants were breastfed, and complementary foods were offered as they got older. Children were from Brazil, Norway, Ghana, Oman, India, and the United States, with careful attention paid to ensure children included in the sample had environmental conditions that would support normal growth to reach their genetic potential. Longitudinal anthropometrics were measured at weeks 1, 2, 4, and 6, monthly from 2 to 12 months, and then bimonthly from 12 to 24 months. Cross-sectional data for children aged 18–71 months was included.

WHO curves demonstrate a faster rate of growth for the first 3 months, followed by slower gains when compared to CDC curves. Infants who are breastfed tend to follow WHO curves, with an initial period of more robust growth followed by deceleration of their growth velocity. Breastfed infants exhibiting normal growth following this pattern may have appeared to be failing to grow appropriately if plotted on CDC charts resulting in unnecessary formula supplementation in breastfed infants. WHO curves have led to lower rates of underweight-for-age and overweight-for-length diagnoses. All patients who fall below the third percentile on WHO growth curves should undergo evaluation for poor growth. WHO curves are therefore the recommended growth standard for assessment of infants up until 2 years of age in the United States.

In summary, AAP recommendations in the United States are to use WHO growth charts until 24 months of age, and then CDC growth charts from 2 to 20 years of age [1]. Use WHO charts from birth for infants born full-term at 37 weeks or greater, and for preterm infants once they are above 41 weeks corrected age. Infants born prior to 37 weeks gestation would appear inaccurately low on the WHO curve based on their actual age instead of their gestational age, and the WHO study populations do not reflect preterm infants. They merit the use of specialized preterm growth charts to assess their postnatal growth prior to reaching term corrected age.

Preterm Growth Charts

The goal for growth in preterm infants is to replicate intrauterine growth velocity at their current gestational age. However, while neonatology has accomplished incredible breakthroughs in caring for premature infants, the postnatal environment does not match the ideal circumstances for growth provided in utero. Therefore, infants born preterm are unlikely to achieve growth congruent with that of healthy fetuses in utero. Intrauterine growth curves are prescriptive, describing ideal growth for a premature infant's corresponding gestational age. Additionally, while ultrasound allows estimation of intrauterine growth, there is no way to measure actual fetal weight in utero. Birth weight of premature infants may correspond with intrauterine weights at those respective weeks of gestation; yet various risk factors that may contribute to intrauterine growth restriction, preterm labor, prematurity, and being born small for gestational age may be confounding in preterm infants and not in infants born at term. The purpose of preterm postnatal curves is to assess growth of a preterm infant compared to growth of other preterm infants and serve as another tool to use along with intrauterine growth curves. The Olsen and Fenton curves are used to assess anthropometrics at birth and subsequent growth of preterm infants until 41 and 50 weeks corrected age, respectively.

In 1966, Lubchenco et al. published descriptive growth curves made from birth measurements of infants born at 26–42 weeks gestation and in 1976 Babson and Benda published growth charts that went from 26 weeks post-menstrual age through 12 months corrected age [38]. This was done by combining intrauterine and postnatal growth data to allow continued follow-up growth of infants born preterm. At that time, the definition of LBW as less than 2500 g was agreed upon by the World Health Assembly [39]. Over time, advancements in neonatal resuscitation and intensive care of premature infants improved, leading to increased survival of smaller LBW infants. Therefore VLBW was defined as less than 1500 g and ELBW as less than 1000 g at birth, regardless of the number of weeks gestation at birth. To account for weeks of gestation completed at birth, in 1995 WHO defined small for gestational age (SGA) as being less than the 10th percentile, appropriate for gestational age (AGA) as being between the 10th and 90th percentiles, and large for gestational age (LGA) as being greater than the 90th percentile for infants of their own gender born at the same gestational age. Table 3.5 lists these definitions. Birth weight, length, and head circumference can each be classified in terms of appropriateness for gestational age and sex by plotting each anthropometric measurement on its respective curve [42].

The transition from following infants on the preterm curves to standard curves once they reached term corrected age was disjointed given that the curves were contiguous with one another. Postnatal curves for preterm infants were first developed by Guo et al. who published curves for weight, length, and head circumference through the first 3 years of life in 1997 [43]. In 1999, Ehrenkranz et al. published postnatal curves for VLBW and ELBW preterm infants based on a cohort of preterm infants with a birth weight of 501–1501 g born in 1994–1995 and then followed postnatally [44]. Most VLBW infants did not achieve catch-up growth during their hospitalization prior to reaching term corrected age when compared with intrauterine growth rates. In 2003, Fenton et al. published unisex growth curves with data from 22 to 50 weeks post-menstrual age from eight countries. This allowed assessment of appropriateness for gestational age of infants born at less than 23 weeks gestation and those that LBW, VLBW, and ELBW with birth weight <2 kg.

In 2010, Olsen et al. published sex-specific curves for infants born 23–41 weeks post-menstrual age (PMA). The Olsen data is a stronger dataset—drawn from actual measurements from 1998 to 2006 of a larger group of ~250,000 racially diverse children in the United States. This data allows following of an infant's growth from 23 to 41 weeks PMA and then ends at term (41 weeks). Using the validated dataset for the 2010 publication on weight-for-age, length-for-age, and head circumference-for-age curves, 2015 Olsen charts include BMI-for-age curves for preterm infants. These BMI curves are for adjunctive use with the other curves to identify and qualify disproportionate growth, and should not be used alone to assess nutritional status.

TABLE 3.5 Weight gain velocity from 2 weeks to 2 years of age. This table contains median weight gain goals to maintain growth percentiles. If a patient is gaining less than 25% of the medial goal weight gain per day, the diagnosis of severe malnutrition can be made; if less than 50%, moderate malnutrition, and if <75% of median goal weight gain per day is gained, severe malnutrition can be diagnosed, respectively. Individual patient goals may need adjustment. Table adapted from the CHOP Clinical Pathway for Infant Malnutrition [37] https://www.chop.edu/clinical-pathway/infant-malnutrition-ftt-assess-growth-and-severity-malnutrition, WHO Child Growth Standards July 2010 (25th–75th%) [40], and Fomon et al. [41]

Age (corrected for prematurity)	Median expected weight gain (g/day)	
Sex	Girls	Boys
2–4 weeks	29	34
4 weeks–2 months	34	40
2–3 months	24	27
3–4 months	20	21
4–5 months	16	17
5–6 months	13	14
6–8 months	11	11
8–10 months	9	8
10–12 months	9	8
12–18 months	7	7
18–24 months	7	6

Average weight gain requirement of VLBW infants						
Body weight	500–700 g	700–900 g	900–1200 g	1200–1500 g	1500–1800 g	1800–2200 g
Weight gain goal	21 g/kg/day	20 g/kg/day	19 g/kg/day	18 g/kg/day	16 g/kg/day	14 g/kg/day

Revised Fenton charts that are more robust and sex-specific were published in 2013. They harmonized multiple datasets including the Olsen data and new WHO growth standards by smoothing curves while maintaining data integrity between 22 to 36 weeks, and at 50 weeks. This allows preterm infants born at 22 weeks gestation or greater to be followed on the same curve from birth until 50 weeks and beyond, supporting the continuity of growth assessment. It is our practice to use the Olsen charts at birth for all newborns born at 23 weeks or greater to assess appropriateness for gestational age of birth weight, length, and head circumference. Fenton charts are used for those born at less than 23 weeks since Fenton curves start at 22 weeks.

To determine appropriateness for gestational age in all neonates, plot birth measurements on the Olsen or Fenton curves based on their gestational age. Free electronic tools are available to facilitate this assessment such as http://www.Peditools.org and the PediTools: Fenton 2013 application. Enter a newborn's date of birth and gestational age along with birth weight, height, and/or head circumference, and each value is plotted on its respective curve providing a visual representation of where they fall compared to other infants and whether they are SGA, AGA, or LGA, respectively. See Table 3.6 for a summary of growth charts recommended for use. Use Olsen 2010 or Fenton 2013 charts to assess birth anthropometrics in all neonates, as well as to assess postnatal growth in all preterm infants. Once preterm infants have reached 41–50 weeks of corrected gestational age, use WHO curves.

Diagnosis-Specific Growth Charts

Growth charts exist for patients with specific diagnoses based on descriptive data, such as those for achondroplasia, Trisomy 21, Turner Syndrome, and Williams syndrome. See Table 3.7

TABLE 3.6 Assessment of birth anthropometrics

Classification	Definition
Low birth weight (LBW)	Birth weight < 2500 g
Very low birth weight (VLBW)	Birth weight < 1500 g
Extremely low birth weight (ELBW)	Birthweight <1000 g
Small for gestational age (SGA)	<10th percentile for gestational age
Appropriate for gestational age (AGA)	Between the 10th and 90th percentile for gestational age
Large for gestational age (LGA)	>90th percentile for gestational age

for a list of several conditions with published growth charts. Some of the sample sizes used in creating these charts were small and therefore the charts may not be representative of all patients with these diagnoses. Most of these specialty growth charts are descriptive, other than the weight charts for cerebral palsy (CP), which have some prescriptive qualities and were first published in 2007 by Day et al. and then updated in 2011 by Brooks et al. [48, 49]. There are five different curves based on gross motor function score (GMFCS) I, II, III, IV, and V [49]. GMFCS V represent children who are wheelchair-bound and non-ambulatory. Level V is subdivided into children who are tube fed (TF) or not tube fed (NT). The charts can be found on the website http://www.lifeexpectancy.org/articles/GrowthCharts.shtml and http://www.lifeexpectancy.org/articles/NewGrowthCharts/All.pdf [49]. The red shaded area on the charts is indicative of a "danger zone" and patients who plot in this area are at risk for increased morbidity and mortality. The study did not evaluate Z-scores to diagnose malnutrition, so the CP charts can be used to support or refute a diagnosis of malnutrition in conjunction with other malnutrition criteria such as weight loss.

TABLE 3.7 Growth charts: types and interpretation

Growth chart	Age range	Year published	Type of growth charts and comments
Olsen [45]	≥23 weeks at birth through 41 weeks completed	2010, 2015	Recumbent length, weight, HC, and BMI-for-age [46]
Fenton [47]	≥22 weeks at birth through 50 weeks of age	2003, 2013	Actual age (vs. weeks completed) sex-specific ideal goal growth for the fetus, preterm infant, followed by term infant; allows appropriateness for GA to be assessed in infants <2 kg
WHO [2]	≥37 weeks at birth and preterm corrected >41 weeks through 24 months	2006	Recumbent length, weight, weight-for-length, and HC-for-age
CDC [3]	2–20 years	2000	Standing height, weight, and BMI-for-age; alternative height measurements (described in Table 3.2) can be plotted on CDC height curves
Obesity extension curves [36]	2–20 years	2017	Curves for >120% (class 2 obesity) and >140% (class 3 obesity) of CDC 95th percentile [36]

Brooks et al. concluded that children with CP who have very low weights have more major medical conditions and are at increased risk of death [49]. Patients with CP above the

20th percentile for weight-for-age on the new CP charts in GMFCS levels I–IV and V without feeding tubes had less morbidity and mortality ($p < 0.01$). Weight below the fifth percentile for GMFCS levels I and II was associated with a mortality hazard ratio of 2.2 (95% confidence interval: 1.3–3.7) [49]. For children in GMFCS levels III through V, weight below the 20th percentile was associated with a mortality hazard ratio of 1.5 (95% confidence interval: 1.4–1.7) [49].

There are recently published BMI extension curves for patients over the 95th percentile on the CDC curve, which allows diagnosis of classes 1, 2, and 3 obesity [36]. See Table 3.4.

Plotting Growth Measurements

For growth assessment to be accurate, each measurement (weight, length/height, and head circumference) and weight-for-length or BMI must be plotted on the clinically appropriate growth chart to avoid misclassification of growth status. Many electronic health records have the capability to plot measurements on growth charts, and many allow the user to input historical data points from other institutions. Alternatively, measurements can be plotted by hand on printed growth charts or on Peditools.org to generate curves electronically. It is important to plot and track growth over time. Multiple longitudinal measurements allow comparison and assessment of growth trends of a patient over time compared to their own individual growth history and to their clinically appropriate reference population for age.

Plot measurements of preterm infants for their corrected age (number of weeks they were born prior to term subtracted from their chronological age) after they have reached term until at least 24–36 months [1]. After that, there should no longer be major growth differences compared to children born full-term, although there may still be some variation and some are proponents of using a corrected age through 7 years of age. Growth charts in electronic health records may allow correction for gestational age, some with a visual representation of the shifting of the curves from being plotted for chronological versus corrected age.

Interpretation

Newborns lose weight during the first few days of life because of fluid shifts, metabolic changes, thermic effect of food, and increased energy needs for adaptation. After 3–5 days and no later than 7 days of life, the weight loss should resolve and birthweight recover by 2 weeks of age. After this period, for the first 2 months of life, weight gain and linear growth velocity are at their lifetime peak. See Table 3.8 for median goal weight gain velocity based on age [6]. The peak linear growth velocity is almost 1 cm per week through 4 months of age. Each week, infants gain 0.8–0.93 cm in length per week, which adds up to 3.47–4.03 cm per month, and after 4 months, linear growth velocity slows progressively with age [80].

Infants require calories to fuel their metabolism and energy expenditure, and weight gain is a marker of adequate caloric intake. Linear growth will only occur if there is a positive energy balance. Therefore, weight gain occurs first and linear growth happens after a period of sufficient weight gain. This results in growth spurts usually in a stepladder fashion. When patients are not growing adequately, their height accrual may decelerate. Decline in the slope of a height curve may be subtle and less obvious in the early stages. In general, weight falls off before length; and the last parameter to suffer is the head circumference. As a general guideline, children should grow at least 5 cm per year. If not, they merit referral to an endocrinologist. Height velocity curves are part of an endocrinologist's evaluation.

Children tend to shift from their birth trajectory to their own track on the growth chart between 9 and 18 months of age and therefore crossing percentiles or Z-scores can be normal during this age range. This is due to the natural process of adjusting from the track of their in utero growth,

TABLE 3.8 Specialty growth charts: diagnosis-specific descriptive growth charts

Diagnosis	Most recent year published
22q11 Deletion (DiGeorge, Velocardiofacial syndrome) [50, 51]	2012
Achondroplasia (Horton, Rotter, Rimoin, Scott, and Hall, 1978) and Diastrophic dysplasia, spondyloepiphyseal dysplasia congenita, pseudoachondroplasia [52, 53]	1978
Cerebral palsy [48, 49]	2011
Congenital adrenal hyperplasia (classical 21-hydroxylase deficiency) [54]	1998
Cornelia de Lange Syndrome [55]	1993
Costello Syndrome [56]	2012
Duchene's Muscular Dystrophy [57–59]	1988
Ellis–van Creveld syndrome [60]	2010
Klinefelter's Syndrome (47, XXY) [61]	1974
Marfan Syndrome [62]	2002
Myelomeningocele [63, 64]	1999
Neurofibromatosis type 1 [65]	1999
Noonan Syndrome [66, 67]	2017
Obesity extension curves (severe class 2 and 3 obesity) [36]	2017
Osteogenesis Imperfecta type 1 [68]	2017
Prader Willi Syndrome [69, 70]	1988
Rett Syndrome [71]	2012
Rubinstein-Taybi syndrome [72]	2014
Shwachman Diamond [73]	2019

(continued)

Table 3.8 (continued)

Diagnosis	Most recent year published
Silver-Russell Syndrome [74]	1995
Trisomy 21 (Down Syndrome) [75]	2015
Turner Syndrome (45, XO) [36, 67]	2017
Williams-Beuren Syndrome [76–79]	2004

based on their mother's nutritional status during gestation and placental sufficiency, to their postnatal growth track, based on their genetic potential and influenced by their environmental energy intake and expenditure.

In children and adolescents, linear growth is an important anthropometric and surrogate marker for bone accrual [81]. When interpreting height, pubertal status assessment using Tanner staging is important. This helps determine growth potential and identify pubertal delays. Udry et al. showed that self-assessment of Tanner staging correlates with pubertal changes [82].

To assess linear growth, compare the length or height to a patient's previous stature, age and sex-related normative data, sexual maturity, and to estimate genetic potential stature based on the stature of each parent. Mid-parental height is useful to estimate the growth potential of a child based on the height of their parents. Comparing a patient's stature to their calculated mid-parental height is a way to identify growth failure compared to their own genetic background. In 1970, Tanner and Whitehead described a method of estimating height potential by calculating mid-parental height, and these equations were updated in 1986 by Falkner & Tanner [29, 83].

Percent ideal body weight for height via the McLaren or Moore method was historically a part of growth assessment based on height age, influenced by age and puberty [84, 85]. Ideal body weight has limitations in that it assumes that children at the 50th percentile for height have a mean weight at the 50th percentile for weight. This assumes that percentile

TABLE 3.9 Growth and malnutrition clinical pathways from CHOP

Clinical pathway for identification and diagnosis of inpatient pediatric malnutrition (undernutrition) [37] https://www.chop.edu/clinical-pathway/malnutrition-undernutrition-clinical-pathway
Clinical pathway for infant and pediatric outpatient malnutrition Management [86]. https://www.chop.edu/clinical-pathway/infant-malnutrition-outpatient-specialty-care-and-primary-care-clinical-pathway
Inpatient clinical pathway for evaluation/treatment of infants with malnutrition (failure to thrive) <12 month [87] https://www.chop.edu/clinical-pathway/infant-malnutrition-ftt-clinical-pathway
Outpatient clinical pathway for obesity prevention and Management [88] https://www.chop.edu/clinical-pathway/obesity-prevention-and-management-clinical-pathway

Available Online (Open Access)

distributions for height correspond to the percentile distributions for weight and do not reflect real height–weight combinations of children. We have moved away from using this tool since the weight–height relationship is complex.

Clinical pathways created in groups such as ours provide resources and recommendations for growth measurements including plotting on growth charts, monitoring, interpreting, and treating malnutrition (overnutrition or undernutrition) if present. Table 3.9 shows some of the available CHOP clinical pathways for growth assessment and malnutrition with links to access them.

Malnutrition Diagnosis Criteria

Criteria for diagnosing malnutrition and its severity vary by age. There are no defined malnutrition criteria for infants less than 7 days old since it is normal to lose less than 15% of birth weight in the first days of life. From 7 to 14 days of life, and 15 days to 1 month, there are specific malnutrition diagnosis criteria shown in Table 3.10. After the first month, his-

TABLE 3.10 Diagnosis of pediatric malnutrition and severity <1 month corrected Age

Age	Indicators	Malnutrition diagnosis severity			Notes for use
		Severe	Moderate	Mild	
7–14 days old	Nutrient intake ≤ 75% of needs	>7 days (consecutive)	≥5–7 days (consecutive)	≥3–5 days (consecutive)	Estimated calorie needs by age
15 days to 1 month corrected age	Weight gain velocity	<25% of expected	<50% of expected	<75% of expected	Preterm: Use *Peditools.org* Term: Use Table 3.4
	Weight-for-age Z-score decline	>2 SD decline	1.21–2 SD decline	0.8–1.2 SD decline	*Peditools.org* for accurate Z-score
	Days to regain birth weight	>21	19–21	15–18	Must use with nutrient intake indicator

>1 month corrected age to 18 years of age

Indicators	Malnutrition diagnosis severity		
	Severe	Moderate	Mild
Weight for height (1–24 mos)	≤ −3 Z-score	−2.0 to −2.99 Z-score	−1.0 to −1.99 Z-score[a]
Weight gain velocity (≤24 mos)	≤25% of normal	<50% of normal	<75% of the normal
Mid-upper arm circumference[b]	≤−3 Z-score	−2.0 to −2.99 Z-score	−1.0 to −1.99 Z-score
BMI-for-age (>2 yrs)	≤ − 3 Z-score	−2.0 to −2.99 Z-score	−1.0 to −1.99 Z-score[a]
Weight loss (>2 yrs)	>10% of weight	>7.5% of weight	>5% of weight
Length/height Z-score	≤−3 Z-score	No data available	No data available
Deceleration in Wt for Ht; BMI	Decline of 3 Z-score	Decline of 2 Z-score	Decline of 1 Z-score
Inadequate nutrient intake	≤25% of estimated energy/protein need	26–50% of estimated energy/protein need	51–75% of estimated energy/protein need

SD Standard Deviation, *mos* months, *Wt for Ht* weight for length/height for age, *yrs* years

[a]Needs additional positive diagnostic criteria for diagnosis

[b]MUAC suggested between 6–60 months. If a child meets more than one malnutrition acuity level, the provider should document the severity of the malnutrition at the highest acuity level met to ensure appropriate monitoring, evaluation, intervention, and treatment

Table adapted from CHOP Clinical Pathways for Pediatric Malnutrition [37]

https://www.chop.edu/clinical-pathway/infant-malnutrition-ftt-assess-growth-and-severity-malnutrition

https://www.chop.edu/clinical-pathway/malnutrition-undernutrition-comprehensive-malnutrition-indicators-table

torically there have been multiple definitions used to diagnose malnutrition, e.g., WHO and Waterloo-based on growth chart percentiles. Z-scores are now used as they provide more information than percentiles or absolute number measurements. In 2015, the American Society for Parenteral and Enteral Nutrition (ASPEN) and the Academy of Nutrition and Dietetics (AND) defined malnutrition for children older than 1 month corrected age to 18 years of age. Z-scores for weight for length/height (<2 years) or BMI-for-age (>2 years), mid-upper arm circumference for age, or deceleration of one of those Z-scores can be sufficient alone for a malnutrition diagnosis. Length/height for age Z-scores can also indicate malnutrition but need at least one other indicator to make a diagnosis. The remaining indicators are weight loss, weight gain velocity, and inadequate nutrient intake [89]. In adults >20 years old, BMI classification is based on the BMI number. See Table 3.4 for BMI classification and Table 3.11 for malnutrition diagnosis criteria in adults. When length and weight are not available, Kanawati et al. described using the ratio of mid-upper arm circumference: head circumference in young children up to 3 years old. A ratio >0.31 is normal and <0.25 indicates severe malnutrition [84].

TABLE 3.11 Adult malnutrition (19+ years of age)

Malnutrition level	Moderate			Severe		
Illness/injury	Acute	Chronic	Social/environment	Acute	Chronic	Social/environment
Reduced food intake	<75%>7 days	<75%>30 days	<75%>90 days	<50%>5 days	<75%>30 days	<50%>30 days
Weight loss	1–2%, 1 week			>2%, 1 week		
	5%, 1 month			>5%, 1 month		
	7.5%, 3 months			>7.5%, 3 months		
	10%, 6 months			>10%, 6 months		
	20%, 1 year			>20%, 1 year		
Fat loss	Mild			Moderate	Severe	Severe
Muscle loss	Mild			Moderate	Severe	Severe

The selection of two or more criteria is required for a moderate or severe malnutrition evaluation

Table adapted table from Consensus Statement of the Academy of Nutrition and Dietetics/American Society for Parenteral and Enteral Nutrition: Characteristics Recommended for the Identification and Documentation of Adult Malnutrition (Undernutrition) [89] and the CHOP pathway for Malnutrition [37]

https://www.chop.edu/clinical-pathway/malnutrition-undernutrition-comprehensive-malnutrition-indicators-table

Intervention

Red flags pointing toward the need for evaluation and intervention in children with failure to thrive/faltering growth include lack of appropriate weight gain. In normal newborn development, weight loss stops by day 5 and no later than day 7 of life, with the recovery of birthweight by 2–3 weeks of life. If weight loss continues beyond day 5 or they have not regained birthweight by 21 days, that is concerning [1]. If patients' Z-scores for height and weight are abnormal, or if their Z-scores are crossing Z-score lines representing standard deviations for age, this is concerning. This is the equivalent of dropping growth percentiles and crossing percentile lines on growth charts. Delayed bone age for chronological age based on the Greulich and Pyle or Tanner–Whitehouse method is a red flag [10]. When height is not within range of normal for age, it is important to compare the patient's linear growth to their genetic potential based on their projected mid-parental height, pursuing further evaluation when their progress is not on target. Signs or symptoms suggestive of underlying organic disease are also concerning, such as dehydration, abnormal vital signs, or wasting of subcutaneous fat stores on exam. Infants who feed less than 8 times, have less than 6–8 wet diapers in 1 day, are lethargic, or are not passing meconium or stool also warrant further work up. In the first year of life, weight loss or lack of appropriate weight gain is abnormal. Infants and children should be gaining and following the trend of weight for their age. If a child loses more than 5% of their body weight, it is a warning sign and more than 10% is a red flag. Severe malnutrition is present when weight-for-length or BMI have a Z-score of −3 (or farther from the mean) [89].

If a patient is not growing, the most important thing to do first is to repeat the growth measurements and make sure they are measured, reported, and recorded correctly, as well as plotted correctly on the appropriate growth chart. Poor growth is due to inadequate caloric intake, inadequate caloric absorption/utilization, or increased caloric requirement. Inadequate intake is the most common cause of poor growth and failure to thrive in infants and children. It is important to observe feeding and provide emotional cues and caregiver relationship in an accepting and nonjudgmental way, as caregivers can sometimes self-blame themselves for their infant's poor growth. Evaluation by a registered dietitian, feeding specialists, pediatric gastroenterologist, and other health care professionals may be helpful.

Conclusion

Growth assessment is an important part of the care of all infants, children, and adolescents. Accurate measurements, use of the correct growth charts, and interpretation of the data are key points in assessing nutritional status and developing appropriate and specific interventions.

References

1. Kleinman RE, Greer FR, eds. Pediatric Nutrition. American Academy of Pediatrics. 2013. https://doi.org/10.1542/9781610023610.
2. de Onis M, Garza C, Onyango AW, Rolland-Cachera MF. WHO growth standards for infants and young children. Arch Pediatr. 2009;16(1):47–53.
3. Kuczmarski RJ, Ogden CL, Grummer-Strawn LM, et al. CDC growth charts: United States. Adv Data. 2000;314:1–27.
4. Nellhaus G. Head circumference from birth to eighteen years. Practical composite international and interracial graphs. Pediatrics. 1968;41(1):106–14.
5. Lipman TH, Cousounis P, Grundmeier RW, et al. Electronic health record mid-parental height auto-calculator for growth assessment in primary care. Clin Pediatr (Phila). 2016;55(12):1100–6.
6. Danner E, Joeckel R, Michalak S, Phillips S, Goday PS. Weight velocity in infants and children. Nutr Clin Pract. 2009;24(1):76–9.
7. Fenton TR, Senterre T, Griffin IJ. Time interval for preterm infant weight gain velocity calculation precision. Arch Dis Child Fetal Neonatal Ed. 2019;104(2):F218–f219.

8. Berkey CS, Dockery DW, Wang X, Wypij D, Ferris B Jr. Longitudinal height velocity standards for U.S. adolescents. Stat Med. 1993;12(3–4):403–14.

9. Anderson M. Use of the Greulich-Pyle "atlas of skeletal development of the hand and wrist" in a clinical context. Am J Phys Anthropol. 1971;35(3):347–52.

10. Bull RK, Edwards PD, Kemp PM, Fry S, Hughes IA. Bone age assessment: a large scale comparison of the Greulich and Pyle, and Tanner and Whitehouse (TW2) methods. Arch Dis Child. 1999;81(2):172–3.

11. Milner GR, Levick RK, Kay R. Assessment of bone age: a comparison of the Greulich and Pyle, and the Tanner and Whitehouse methods. Clin Radiol. 1986;37(2):119–21.

12. Bayley N, Pinneau SR. Tables for predicting adult height from skeletal age: revised for use with the Greulich-Pyle hand standards. J Pediatr. 1952;40(4):423–41.

13. de Onis M, Garza C, Onyango AW, Borghi E. Comparison of the WHO child growth standards and the CDC 2000 growth charts. J Nutr. 2007;137(1):144–8.

14. Stevenson RD. Use of segmental measures to estimate stature in children with cerebral palsy. Arch Pediatr Adolesc Med. 1995;149(6):658–62.

15. Hibbert ME, Lanigan A, Raven J, Phelan PD. Relation of armspan to height and the prediction of lung function. Thorax. 1988;43(8):657–9.

16. Gauld LM, Kappers J, Carlin JB, Robertson CF. Height prediction from ulna length. Dev Med Child Neurol. 2004;46(7):475–80.

17. Hogan SE. Knee height as a predictor of recumbent length for individuals with mobility-impaired cerebral palsy. J Am Coll Nutr. 1999;18(2):201–5.

18. Bell KL, Davies PS. Prediction of height from knee height in children with cerebral palsy and non-disabled children. Ann Hum Biol. 2006;33(4):493–9.

19. Chumlea WMC, Guo SS, Steinbaugh ML. Prediction of stature from knee height for black and white adults and children with application to mobility-impaired or handicapped persons. J Am Diet Assoc. 1994;94(12):1385–91.

20. Kihara K, Kawasaki Y, Yagi M, Takada S. Relationship between stature and tibial length for children with moderate-to-severe cerebral palsy. Brain Dev. 2015;37(9):853–7.

21. Oeffinger D, Conaway M, Stevenson R, Hall J, Shapiro R, Tylkowski C. Tibial length growth curves for ambulatory chil-

dren and adolescents with cerebral palsy. Dev Med Child Neurol. 2010;52(9):e195–201.

22. Hamill PV, et al. Body weight, stature, and sitting height. US Vital and Health Statistics, Series 11, #126; Publication No HSM 73–1606. Washington, DC: US Government Printing Office; 1973.

23. Reilly JJ. Determination from body composition from skinfold thickness: a validation study. Arch Dis Child. 1995;73:305–10.

24. Addo OY, Himes JH, Zemel BS. Reference ranges for midupper arm circumference, upper arm muscle area, and upper arm fat area in US children and adolescents aged 1-20 y. Am J Clin Nutr. 2017;105(1):111–20.

25. Frisancho AR. New norms of upper limb fat and muscle areas for assessment of nutritional status. Am J Clin Nutr. 1981;34(11):2540–5.

26. Addo OY, Himes JH. Reference curves for triceps and subscapular skinfold thicknesses in US children and adolescents. Am J Clin Nutr. 2010;91(3):635–42.

27. Wellens R, Roche AF, Guo S, Chumlea WC, Siervogel RM. Fat-free mass and percent body fat assessments by dual-energy X-ray absorptiometry, densitometry and total body water. Basic Life Sci. 1993;60:71–4.

28. Mazess RB, Barden HS, Bisek JP, Hanson J. Dual-energy x-ray absorptiometry for total-body and regional bone-mineral and soft-tissue composition. Am J Clin Nutr. 1990;51(6):1106–12.

29. Tanner JM. 1 Normal growth and techniques of growth assessment. Clin Endocrinol Metab. 1986;15(3):411–51.

30. Durnin JV, Rahaman MM. The assessment of the amount of fat in the human body from measurements of skinfold thickness. Br J Nutr. 1967;21(3):681–9.

31. Wendel D, Weber D, Leonard MB, et al. Body composition estimation using skinfolds in children with and without health conditions affecting growth and body composition. Ann Hum Biol. 2017;44(2):108–20.

32. Brook CG. Determination of body composition of children from skinfold measurements. Arch Dis Child. 1971;46(246):182–4.

33. McDowell I, King FS. Interpretation of arm circumference as an indicator of nutritional status. Arch Dis Child. 1982;57(4):292–6.

34. Weber DR, Boyce A, Gordon C, et al. The utility of DXA assessment at the forearm, proximal femur, and lateral distal femur, and vertebral fracture assessment in the pediatric population: 2019 ISCD official position. J Clin Densitom. 2019;22(4):567–89.

35. Crabtree NJ, Arabi A, Bachrach LK, et al. Dual-energy X-ray absorptiometry interpretation and reporting in children and adolescents: the revised 2013 ISCD pediatric official positions. J Clin Densitom. 2014;17(2):225–42.
36. Racette SB, Yu L, DuPont NC, Clark BR. BMI-for-age graphs with severe obesity percentile curves: tools for plotting cross-sectional and longitudinal youth BMI data. BMC Pediatr. 2017;17(1):130.
37. Smith E, Weston S, Dean A, et al. Clinical pathway for identification and diagnosis of inpatient pediatric malnutrition (undernutrition). The Children's Hospital of Philadelphia Clinical Pathway Program. Malnutrition pathways web site. https://www.chop.edu/clinical-pathway/malnutrition-undernutrition-clinical-pathway. Published March 2016. Updated March 2018. Accessed 2020.
38. Babson SG, Benda GI. Growth graphs for the clinical assessment of infants of varying gestational age. J Pediatr. 1976;89(5):814–20.
39. Cutland CL, Lackritz EM, Mallett-Moore T, et al. Low birth weight: Case definition & guidelines for data collection, analysis, and presentation of maternal immunization safety data. Vaccine. 2017;35(48 Pt A):6492–500.
40. Grummer-Strawn LM, Reinold C, Krebs NF. Centers for disease C, prevention. Use of World Health Organization and CDC growth charts for children aged 0-59 months in the United States. MMWR Recomm Rep. 2010;59(RR-9):1–15.
41. Fomon SJ, Haschke F, Ziegler EE, Nelson SE. Body composition of reference children from birth to age 10 years. Am J Clin Nutr. 1982;35(5 Suppl):1169–75.
42. Lubchenco LO, Hansman C, Boyd E. Intrauterine growth in length and head circumference as estimated from live births at gestational ages from 26 to 42 weeks. Pediatrics. 1966;37(3):403–8.
43. Guo SS, Roche AF, Chumlea WC, Casey PH, Moore WM. Growth in weight, recumbent length, and head circumference for preterm low-birthweight infants during the first three years of life using gestation-adjusted ages. Early Hum Dev. 1997;47(3):305–25.
44. Ehrenkranz RA, Younes N, Lemons JA, et al. Longitudinal growth of hospitalized very low birth weight infants. Pediatrics. 1999;104(2 Pt 1):280–9.
45. Olsen IE, Groveman SA, Lawson ML, Clark RH, Zemel BS. New intrauterine growth curves based on United States data. Pediatrics. 2010;125(2):e214–24.

46. Olsen IE, Lawson ML, Ferguson AN, et al. BMI curves for preterm infants. Pediatrics. 2015;135(3):e572–81.

47. Fenton TR, Kim JH. A systematic review and meta-analysis to revise the Fenton growth chart for preterm infants. BMC Pediatr. 2013;13:59.

48. Day SM, Strauss DJ, Vachon PJ, Rosenbloom L, Shavelle RM, Wu YW. Growth patterns in a population of children and adolescents with cerebral palsy. Dev Med Child Neurol. 2007;49(3):167–71.

49. Brooks J, Day S, Shavelle R, Strauss D. Low weight, morbidity, and mortality in children with cerebral palsy: new clinical growth charts. Pediatrics. 2011;128(2):e299–307.

50. Habel A, McGinn M-J II, Zackai EH, Unanue N, McDonald-McGinn DM. Syndrome-specific growth charts for 22q11.2 deletion syndrome in Caucasian children. Am J Med Genet A. 2012;158A(11):2665–71.

51. Tarquinio DC, Jones MC, Jones KL, Bird LM. Growth charts for 22q11 deletion syndrome. Am J Med Genet A. 2012;158a(11):2672–81.

52. Horton WA, Hall JG, Scott CI, Pyeritz RE, Rimoin DL. Growth curves for height for diastrophic dysplasia, spondyloepiphyseal dysplasia congenita, and pseudoachondroplasia. Am J Dis Child. 1982;136(4):316–9.

53. Horton WA, Rotter JI, Rimoin DL, Scott CI, Hall JG. Standard growth curves for achondroplasia. J Pediatr. 1978;93(3):435–8.

54. Hargitai G, Sólyom J, Battelino T, et al. Growth patterns and final height in congenital adrenal hyperplasia due to classical 21-hydroxylase deficiency. Horm Res Paediatr. 2001;55(4):161–71.

55. Kline AD, Barr M, Jackson LG. Growth manifestations in the Brachmann-de Lange syndrome. Am J Med Genet. 1993;47(7):1042–9.

56. Sammon MR, Doyle D, Hopkins E, et al. Normative growth charts for individuals with Costello syndrome. Am J Med Genet A. 2012;158a(11):2692–9.

57. Willig TN, Carlier L, Legrand M, Riviere H, Navarro J. Nutritional assessment in Duchenne muscular dystrophy. Dev Med Child Neurol. 1993;35(12):1074–82.

58. Griffiths RD, Edwards RH. A new chart for weight control in Duchenne muscular dystrophy. Arch Dis Child. 1988;63(10):1256–8.

59. Coakley JH, Griffiths RD, Edwards RH. Height and clinical course of Duchenne muscular dystrophy. Am J Med Genet. 1989;32(4):552–4.
60. Verbeek S, Eilers PH, Lawrence K, Hennekam RC, Versteegh FG. Growth charts for children with Ellis-van Creveld syndrome. Eur J Pediatr. 2011;170(2):207–11.
61. Schibler D, Brook CG, Kind HP, Zachmann M, Prader A. Growth and body proportions in 54 boys and men with Klinefelter's syndrome. Helv Paediatr Acta. 1974;29(4):325–33.
62. Erkula G, Jones KB, Sponseller PD, Dietz HC, Pyeritz RE. Growth and maturation in Marfan syndrome. Am J Med Genet. 2002;109(2):100–15.
63. Charney EB, Rosenblum M, Finegold D. Linear growth in a population of children with myelomeningocele. Z Kinderchir. 1981;34(4):415–9.
64. Grogan CB, Ekvall SM. Body composition of children with myelomeningocele, determined by 40K, urinary creatinine and anthropometric measures. J Am Coll Nutr. 1999;18(4):316–23.
65. Clementi M, Milani S, Mammi I, Boni S, Monciotti C, Tenconi R. Neurofibromatosis type 1 growth charts. Am J Med Genet. 1999;87(4):317–23.
66. Witt DR, Keena BA, Hall JG, Allanson JE. Growth curves for height in Noonan syndrome. Clin Genet. 1986;30(3):150–3.
67. Isojima T, Yokoya S. Development of disease-specific growth charts in Turner syndrome and Noonan syndrome. Ann Pediatr Endocrinol Metab. 2017;22(4):240–6.
68. Graff K, Syczewska M. Developmental charts for children with osteogenesis imperfecta, type I (body height, body weight and BMI). Eur J Pediatr. 2017;176(3):311–6.
69. Holm VA, Nugent JK. Growth in the Prader-Willi syndrome. Birth Defects Orig Artic Ser. 1982;18(3b):93–100.
70. Wollmann HA, Schultz U, Grauer ML, Ranke MB. Reference values for height and weight in Prader-Willi syndrome based on 315 patients. Eur J Pediatr. 1998;157(8):634–42.
71. Tarquinio DC, Motil KJ, Hou W, et al. Growth failure and outcome in Rett syndrome: specific growth references. Neurology. 2012;79(16):1653–61.
72. Beets L, Rodriguez-Fonseca C, Hennekam RC. Growth charts for individuals with Rubinstein-Taybi syndrome. Am J Med Genet A. 2014;164a(9):2300–9.

73. Cipolli M, Tridello G, Micheletto A, et al. Normative growth charts for Shwachman-diamond syndrome from Italian cohort of 0–8 years old. BMJ Open. 2019;9(1):e022617.
74. Wollmann HA, Kirchner T, Enders H, Preece MA, Ranke MB. Growth and symptoms in silver-Russell syndrome: review on the basis of 386 patients. Eur J Pediatr. 1995;154(12):958–68.
75. Zemel BS, Pipan M, Stallings VA, et al. Growth charts for children with down syndrome in the United States. Pediatrics. 2015;136(5):e1204–11.
76. Morris CA, Demsey SA, Leonard CO, Dilts C, Blackburn BL. Natural history of Williams syndrome: physical characteristics. J Pediatr. 1988;113(2):318–26.
77. Partsch C-J, Dreyer G, Gosch A, et al. Longitudinal evaluation of growth, puberty, and bone maturation in children with Williams syndrome. J Pediatr. 1999;134(1):82–9.
78. Pankau R, Partsch CJ, Neblung A, Gosch A, Wessel A. Head circumference of children with Williams-Beuren syndrome. Am J Med Genet. 1994;52(3):285–90.
79. Pankau R, Partsch CJ, Gosch A, Oppermann HC, Wessel A. Statural growth in Williams-Beuren syndrome. Eur J Pediatr. 1992;151(10):751–5.
80. Tanner JM, Whitehouse RH. Clinical longitudinal standards for height, weight, height velocity, weight velocity, and stages of puberty. Arch Dis Child. 1976;51(3):170–9.
81. McCormack SE, Cousminer DL, Chesi A, et al. Association between linear growth and bone accrual in a diverse cohort of children and adolescents. JAMA Pediatr. 2017;171(9):e171769.
82. Morris NM, Udry JR. Validation of a self-administered instrument to assess stage of adolescent development. J Youth Adolesc. 1980;9(3):271–80.
83. Tanner JM, Goldstein H, Whitehouse RH. Standards for children's height at ages 2-9 years allowing for heights of parents. Arch Dis Child. 1970;45(244):755–62.
84. Kanawati AA, McLaren DS. Assessment of marginal malnutrition. Nature. 1970;228(5271):573–5.
85. Phillips S, Edlbeck A, Kirby M, Goday P. Ideal body weight in children. Nutr Clin Pract. 2007;22(2):240–5.
86. Goh VM, Owusu-McKenzie J, Voulalas D, et al. Clinical pathway for infant and pediatric outpatient malnutrition management. The Children's Hospital of Philadelphia Clinical Pathway Program 2020.

87. Dunn M, Rasooly I, Brennan B, et al. Inpatient clinical pathway for evaluation/treatment of infants with malnutrition (failure to thrive) < 12 months. The Children's Hospital of Philadelphia Clinical Pathway Program 2019.
88. Khan J, Mascarenhas, M. Outpatient clinical pathway for obesity prevention and management. The Children's Hospital of Philadelphia Clinical Pathway Program 2019.
89. Becker P, Carney LN, Corkins MR, et al. Consensus statement of the academy of nutrition and dietetics/American Society for Parenteral and Enteral Nutrition: indicators recommended for the identification and documentation of pediatric malnutrition (undernutrition). Nutr Clin Pract. 2015;30(1):147–61.

Chapter 4
Management Approach: Enteral Nutrition

Tiffany Williams and Shani Cunningham

The calorie is a *unit of energy* widely used in *nutrition* [1]. In a nutritional context, a calorie is the quantity of heat needed to raise the temperature of 1 kg of water by one degree Celsius [2]. Failure to thrive (FTT) is a state of undernutrition that occurs when caloric intake is insufficient to maintain growth [3].

Nutritional requirements and calorie needs vary widely by age group. Organizations, such as the National Academies of Sciences, Engineering, and Medicine, have developed nutritional reference values, referred to as dietary references intakes (DRIs), which are intended to serve as a guide for proper nutrition and provide the scientific basis for the development of food guidelines in the United States [4]. These nutrient reference values are specified on the basis of age, sex, and special populations (e.g., pregnancy) and cover more than 40 nutrient substances [4]. DRIs are a set of several reference values that are related to both adequate intakes and upper levels of intakes.

T. Williams
Department of Pediatrics, NYU Grossman School of Medicine/
Bellevue Hospital Center, New York, NY, USA

S. Cunningham (✉)
Pediatric Hospital Medicine, AdventHealth for Children,
Orlando, FL, USA
e-mail: Shani.Cunningham.DO@AdventHealth.com

© Springer Nature Switzerland AG 2023
J. G. Vachani (ed.), *Failure to Thrive and Malnutrition*,
https://doi.org/10.1007/978-3-031-14164-5_4

As infants and children attain proper nutrition and caloric intake, most will grow in a predictable fashion, following a typical pattern of progression in weight, length, and head circumference. Term neonates may lose up to 10% of their birth weight in the first few days of life and typically regain their birth weight by 10–14 days [5–8]. Newborns gain approximately 30 g per day (i.e., 1 ounce per day) until 3 months of life. Infants gain approximately 20 g per day (i.e., 0.67 ounces per day) between three and 6 months of life and approximately 10 g per day between 6 and 12 months of life. Additionally, infants double their birth weight by 4 months of life and triple their birth weight by 1 year of life. The growth patterns of preterm infants, small-for-gestational-age infants, and large-for-gestational-age infants differ from these values. Children typically gain approximately 2 kg (i.e., 4.4 pounds) per year between 2 years of life and puberty.

Pediatric evaluation of proper weight gain is vital in order to monitor for and prevent progressive nutritional deficits. Currently, there are several proposed criteria to diagnose FTT [3]. However, all the definitions of FTT require the children to be plotted on an appropriate-for-age growth chart [3]. In 2010, the Centers for Disease Control and Prevention (CDC) recommended that for children younger than 2 years, a World Health Organization (WHO) growth chart should be used, while for children aged 2–19 years, US Centers for Disease Control (CDC) growth chart should instead be used [9]. Special growth charts should be used for children with particular genetic syndromes, such as Down syndrome and Turner syndrome [10].

Pediatric fluid requirements are influenced by factors that include gestational age, postnatal age, disease state, hydration status, environmental temperature and humidity, renal function, insensible water losses, and changes in metabolic rate and respiratory rate. During the first few days of life in newborns, physiologic fluid loss should be anticipated, approximating 2–3% of body weight per day in term infants and 3–5% in preterm infants.

Afterward this period of transition, infants and children generally require at least 115 mL of fluid per 100 kcal of energy provided [11]. Pediatric fluid requirement calculations require correcting for fluid abnormalities (i.e., deficit or excess water) and ongoing maintenance requirements. Excessive loss of fluids such as via gastric output or polyuria must also be measured and replaced. Fluids needed for neutral water balance after accounting for obligatory losses [i.e., maintenance fluid requirements (as further discussed below)] must also be included in fluid requirement calculations.

Pediatric fluids can be given via the enteral or the parenteral route. Enteral nutrition — feeding of nutritional products via the gastrointestinal tract — is preferred, however, a variety of underlying conditions may lead to a need for parenteral nutrition — giving nutritional products intravenously. Initiation of parenteral nutrition is indicated for infants and children whose gastrointestinal tract function is inadequate to support normal growth and development, especially if nutritional support is required for 7 days or more (premature infants and neonates may require earlier intervention) [12]. Additional circumstances for the initiation of parenteral nutrition include: (1) adolescents with short bowel syndrome, (2) long-term congenital diaphragmatic hernia survivors, (3) very low birth weight (VLBW) infants, etc. and other congenital/chronic illnesses [13–15]. The length of time for an infant to achieve full enteral feedings is significantly shorter when parenteral nutrition starts within the first 24 h of life compared to >24 h after birth for VLBW infants [16].

Parenteral nutrition guidelines are based on estimates of maintenance fluid needs, and adjusted for increased or decreased losses as necessary. There are two methods available for the calculation of maintenance of IV fluids in the pediatric population. The first method is The Holliday-Segar method, commonly referred to as the 4-2-1 rule. The second method is the Body Surface Area method, which is calculated based on individual specific body surface area.

The 4-2-1 rule is most commonly used to calculate maintenance fluid needs for healthy children [17]. The 4-2-1 rule can determine the hourly rate of maintenance fluids required for a child based on their weight [18]. The first 10 kg = 4 mL/kg per hour, the next 10–20 kg = 2 mL/kg per hour, and any remaining weight over 20 kg = 1 mL/kg per hour.

For example, a 24-kg child would have the following maintenance fluid requirements:

- First 10 kg = 4 mL/kg per hour × 10 kg = 40 mL per hour
- Next 10–20 kg = 2 mL/kg per hour × 10 kg = 20 mL per hour
- Remaining 4 kg = 1 mL/kg per hour × 2 kg = 4 mL per hour
- Total hourly rate = 40 + 20 + 4 = 64 mL per hour

Special consideration is taken for children who are obese. In such circumstances, the ideal body weight (i.e., 45%ile for height and weight) is used. For children who are not healthy (e.g., dehydrated), the fluids must additionally account for the volume deficit of ongoing losses.

The Body Surface Area (BSA) method can determine the hourly rate of maintenance fluids required for a child based on their height, and hence, their deduced body surface area in square meters. The typical daily requirement is BSA (m^2) 1500–1600 mL/m^2.

For example, a 24-kg child that is 96 cm tall (BSA = 0.8 m^2) would have the following maintenance fluid requirements:

- 0.8 m^2 × 1500 mL/m^2/day
- = 1200 mL/day
- = 1200 mL/day ÷ 24 h/day
- = 50 mL/h

As it is not always feasible to obtain an accurate height in children, such as in children with spasticity or other disorders with contractures making erect stance impractical, the Holliday-Seger method may be more advantageous. Additionally, the Body Surface Area method can only be used for children >3.5 kg.

Enteral nutrition is generally considered the optimal and desirable form of nutrition attainment. In circumstances in which the gastrointestinal tract is only partially functional, if safe to do so, the enteral route should be used even if it is only able to supply a fraction of the required nutrients. There are many different forms of enteral nutrition options (e.g., breast milk and formula). While breastmilk is typically the preferred nutritional option for infants, there are many circumstances and populations for which formula may be the preferred or chosen nutritional option. Many different types of formulas are available for use (Table 4.1).

After selection of an appropriate enteral nutrition formula/breastmilk, nutritional treatment can be optimized by either increasing the total quantity to be consumed or increasing the caloric density (i.e., nutritional enrichment) while maintaining the same total quantity consumed. Many populations benefit from receiving enriched enteral feedings. For example, VLBW infants generally benefit from an enriched diet before and after discharge, especially if there is slow growth or evidence of protein insufficiency or osteopenia during laboratory monitoring [19, 20]. With nutritional enrichment caloric content is increased mainly by either adding carbohydrates and/or fats. Several approaches can be used to enrich the diet based on population characteristics: infant's breastmilk can be fortified (via human milk fortifier, bovine milk-based formula, etc.) or formula can be mixed in such a way to increase the caloric content from the standard 20 kcal/oz. to 22, 24, 27, or more kcal/oz. Other options include the addition of complex carbohydrates (1–3 g/100 mL) and/or oil (grapeseed or sunflower oil, 0.5–1.0 mL/100 mL) [21]. For malabsorption, particularly fat assimilation disorders, adding medium-chain triglycerides (MCTs) can also be beneficial [21]. In small children and school-age children, diet can also be enriched by utilizing puddings, yogurts, and nuts as snacks or by adding cream to sauces and oils to potato or vegetable dishes [21]. Close consultation with a dietitian is recommended to optimize an enteral feeding plan.

Catch-up growth should be monitored closely. Monitoring can be daily, weekly, or monthly depending on the need and

TABLE 4.1 Infant formula comparison chart
Table adapted from Martinez, J. A., & Ballew, M. P. (2011). Infant formulas. Pediatrics in Review, 32 (5), 179–189.
https://doi.org/10.1542/pir.32-5-179

	Primary Protein Source					Carbohydrate						Fat		Features			
	Whey:Casein Ratio	Soy Protein Isolate	Partially Hydrolyzed	Casein Hydrolysate	100% Free Amino Acids	Full Lactose	Reduced Lactose (% Carbohydrate)	Lactose-free	Glucose Polymers	Glucose Polymers/Sucrose Blend	Added Rice Starch (✓) or Soy Fiber (%)	LCT/MCT (%)	DHA/ARA (% total fat)	Osmolality	Nucleotides	Prebiotics	Probiotics
Cow Milk-based Formulas (Intact Protein)																	
Enfamil Premium	60:40					✓						100/0	0.32/0.64	300	✓	✓	
Similac Advance	60:40					✓						100/0	0.15/0.40	310	✓	✓	
Parent's Choice Advantage	60:40								✓			100/0	0.32/0.64	280	✓	✓	
Soy Protein-based Formulas (Intact Protein)																	
Enfamil Prosobee		✓						✓	✓			100/0	0.32/0.64	180			
Similac Sensitive Isomil Soy		✓						✓		✓		100/0	0.15/0.4	200		✓	
Parent's Choice Soy Based		✓					✓	✓	✓			100/0	0.32/0.64	164			
Modified Cow- or Soy Milk-based for Term Infants																	
Enfamil AR	20:80						59%		✓		✓	100/0	0.32/0.64	230			
Enfamil Gentlease	60:40		✓				*20%		✓			100/0	0.32/0.64	230			
Enfamil Restfull	20:80						59%		✓		✓	100/0	0.32/0.64	230			
Good Start Gentle Plus	100:0		✓				70%		✓			100/0	0.32/0.64	250	✓		
Good Start Protect Plus	100:0		✓				70%		✓			100/0	0.32/0.64	250	✓		
Good Start Soy Plus		✓	✓					✓	✓			100/0	0.32/0.64	180			✓
Similac Sensitive	20:80						*trace			✓		100/0	0.15/0.40	200	✓		
Similac Sensitive for Spit-Up	20:80						*trace	✓	✓		✗	100/0	0.15/0.40	180		✓	
Similac Expert Care for Diarrhea									✓			100/0		240	✓		
Parent's Choice Gentle	60:40		✓				25%	✓	✓			100/0	0.32/0.64	189			
Parent's Choice Sensitivity	20:80							✓		✓		100/0	0.32/0.64	198	✓	✓	✓
Parent's Choice Added Rice Starch	20:80						✓		✓		✓	100/0	0.32/0.64	206			
Extensively Hydrolyzed Formulas																	
Nutramigen (liquid concentrate)				✓				✓	✓			100/0	0.32/0.64	260			✓
Nutramigen with Enflora LGG				✓				✓	✓			100/0	0.32/0.64	300			✓
Pregestimil				✓				✓	✓			45/55	0.32/0.64	320			
Similac Expert Care Alimentum				✓				✓		✓		66/33	0.15/0.40	370			
Amino Acid-based Formulas																	
Elecare (unflavored)					✓			✓	✓			67/33	0.15/0/40	350			
Neocate Infant					✓			✓	✓			67/33	0.20/0.35	375			
Nutramigen AA					✓			✓	✓			100/0	0.32/0.64	350			

Milk-based Formulas for Preterm/LBW Infants (RTU 24kcal/oz liquid)															
Enfamil Premature	60-40	-	-	-	-	-	-	-	-	-	60/40	0.32/0.64	300	✓	-
Good Start Premature 24	100:0	-	✓	-	-	-	-	✓	-	-	60/40	0.32/0.40	275	✓✓	-
Similac Special Care 24 Advance	60-40	-	-	-	-	50%	-	✓✓	-	-	50/50	0.25/0.40	280	-	-
Transitional Formulas for Preterm/LBW Infants (RTU 22kcal/oz liquid)															
Enfamil EnfaCare	60-40	-	-	-	-	70%	-	✓	-	-	80/20	0.32/0.64	250	✓✓	-
Similac Expert Care NeoSure	60-40	-	-	-	-	50%	-	✓	-	-	75/25	0.15/0.40	250	✓	-
Cow Milk-based for Specific Medical Needs															
Enfaport (RTU; 30kcal/oz)(for chylothorax; LCHAD)	0:100	-	-	-	-	-	-	✓	-	-	16/84	0.32/0.64	280	-	-
Similac PM (for calcium/phosphorous disorders)	60-40	-	-	✓	-	-	-	-	-	-	100/0	-	280	-	-
Cow Milk-based Follow-Up Formulas (Intact Protein)															
Enfagrow Premium Next Step	20-80	-	-	-	-	55%	-	✓	-	-	100/0	0.32/0.64	270	✓	-
Similac Go and Grow	60-40	-	-	-	-	-	-	✓	-	-	100/0	0.15/0.40	300	✓	-
Parent's Choice Older infants	20-80	-	-	✓	-	71%	-	✓	-	-	100/0	0.32/0.64	282	-	-
Soy Milk-based Follow-Up Formulas (Intact Protein)															
Enfagrow Soy Next Step	-	✓	-	-	-	-	-	✓	-	-	100/0	0.32/0.64	230	-	-
Similac Go and Grow Soy	-	✓	-	-	-	-	-	✓	✓	-	100/0	0.15/0.40	200	-	-
Cow Milk-based Follow-Up Formulas (Modified)															
Enfagrow Gentlease Next Step	60-40	-	-	-	-	*50%	-	✓	-	-	100/0	0.32/0.64	230	-	-
Good Start 2 Gentle Plus	100:0	-	✓	-	-	70%	-	✓	-	-	100/0	0.32/0.64	265	-	-
Parent's Choice Plus	100:0	-	✓	-	-	70%	-	✓	-	-	100/0	0.32/0.64	265	-	✓
Good Start 2 Soy Plus	-	✓	-	-	-	-	-	✓	-	✓	100/0	0.32/0.64	180	-	-

*Formula is marketed for management of "lactose sensitivity."

Enfamil, Prosobee, Nutramigen, Pregestimil, Enfacare, Enfagrow, Enfora, and Enfaport are registered trademark of Mead Johnson Nutrition, Evansville, IN. Patented Natural Defense prebiotic blend used in Enfamil Premium includes galacto-oligosaccharides and polydextrose.

LGG is a trademark of Valio, Ltd.

Good Start, Gentle Plus, Protect Plus, and Soy Plus are registered trademarks of Société des Produits Nestlé S.A., Vevey, Switzerland. Probiotics used in Good Start Protect Plus formulas* *Bifidobacterium lactis.*

Similac, Isomil, Expert Care, Alimentum, Special Care, Neosure, Elecare, and Go and Grow are registered trademarks of Abbott Nutrition, Columbus, OH. Similac Advance contains galacto-oligosaccharides, a prebiotic.

Similac Sensitive Isomil Soy includes fructo-oligosaccharides, a prebiotic.

Parent's Choice is a registered trademark of PBM Nutritionals, Georgia, VT. Parent's Choice Advantage contains galacto-oligosaccharides, a prebiotic.

ARA = arachidonic acid, DHA = docosahexaenoic acid, LBW = low birthweight, LCHAD = long-chain 3-hydroxyacyl-CoA dehydrogenase, LCT = long-chain triglyceride, MCT = medium-chain triglyceride, RTU = ready to use.

severity of illness. You may wish to enlist the help of a registered dietitian to assist with monitoring catch-up growth — either in the inpatient or in the outpatient setting depending on severity of disease, resource availability, and home environment. In infants who are disproportionate in their growth with a length that is in a higher percentage than weight, the ideal body weight can be calculated and placed into the Estimated Energy Requirement Equation (EER) [22]. For infants who are proportionately small, the Scofield equations can be used to calculate the resting metabolic rate (REE) [23], and the REE may then be multiplied by 1.5–2 for catch-up growth [24]. Finally, in small infants where a height may not be available, 110–130 kcal/kg/day is a reasonable estimate for daily requirements [24]. If there are additional considerations, such as cardiac or liver disease, 120–150 kcal/kg/day may be utilized as a starting point [24]. Caloric intake can be adjusted pending weight and overall growth.

While nutritional enrichment and rehabilitation can lead to optimized growth, increased caloric intake can also lead to an altered and suboptimum ratio of calorie, protein, water, and micronutrient intake. If completed quickly and invasively, the swift restoration of caloric intake can pose a risk of life-threatening refeeding syndrome [25, 26]. Refeeding syndrome occurs when a malnourished patient begins to receive adequate nutrition too quickly triggering insulin release and causing intracellular shifts of phosphate, potassium, and magnesium. Although refeeding syndrome is rare except in severe malnutrition, manifestations may include hypophosphatemia (most common), hypokalemia, and hypomagnesemia. Insulin secretion can also cause renal sodium resorption, leading to edema and volume overload. To avoid refeeding syndrome in severely malnourished children, food intake should be increased slowly at first with close consultation with a dietitian and careful monitoring of vital signs, daily weights, strict intake/output, and serum electrolytes [21].

Nutritional enrichment and rehabilitation can be pursued through various means. While the standard form of enteral delivery is via the oral route, there are many circumstances in which this isn't feasible or possible. In such circumstances, a feeding tube may be useful. Feeding tubes are often used in patients whose oral intake is not sufficient to meet their caloric requirements [27]. Some children require long-term enteral access for a variety of medical problems such as failure to thrive in addition to congenital anomalies, inborn errors of metabolism, cystic fibrosis, cerebral palsy, and HIV/AIDS [28].

In nutritional enrichment and rehabilitation, often the most effective way to increase energy intake is to use a feeding tube [21]. When pursuing the use of a feeding tube, there are many possible choices to consider. Least invasive to most invasive common options include a nasogastric (NG) tube, nasoduodenal (ND) tube, nasojejunal (NJ) tube, or a gastrostomy tube (G tube)—which can be further subdivided into a surgical gastrostomy or percutaneous endoscopic gastrostomy (PEG). When choosing a feeding tube, the associated invasiveness and complications must always be considered, as there are benefits and risks to each. Under the guidance of a dietitian, continuous feeds can safely be run through functional feeding tubes; bolus feeds can only be run through nasogastric/gastrostomy tubes (bolus feeds *should not* be given for post-pyloric feeding, i.e., ND or NJ tubes).

1. Nasogastric (NG) tubes: Indicated for a patient whose GI tract is partially or fully functional for nutritional absorption but is unable to maintain adequate oral caloric intake and thus requires short-term nutritional support.
2. Nasoduodenal (ND) tubes: Indicated as described above, and additionally when a patient cannot tolerate NG feeds, such as due to reflux or congenital anomalies.
3. Nasojejunal (NJ) tubes: Indicated as described above, and additionally when a patient cannot tolerate NG or ND feeds, such as due to reflux or congenital anomalies.
4. Surgical gastrostomies (e.g., Gastrostomy (G) tube) [28]: Indicated when a patient has failure to thrive secondary to a variety of medical problems (e.g., cerebral palsy, congenital anomalies, cystic fibrosis, and inborn errors of metabo-

lism) necessitating long-term enteral access for nutritional support. One advantage of surgical gastrostomies, is that for children who cannot tolerate feeds via a G tube, a jejunostomy (J) tube can be placed or their gastrostomy can be converted to a gastrojejunostomy (GJ) tube. For all types, there is a common risk of hypergranulation tissue development. Less commonly, there is a risk of local inflammation, dislocation, aspiration, and faults/obstruction of the tube.

5. Percutaneous endoscopic gastrostomies (PEG) [21, 28]: Indicated when a patient has failure to thrive, secondary to a variety of medical problems (e.g., cerebral palsy, congenital anomalies, cystic fibrosis, and inborn errors of metabolism) necessitating long-term enteral access for nutritional support. One advantage of PEG vs. surgical gastrostomy is that it avoids the risks of general anesthesia. Parents usually prefer PEGs to nasal tubes for long-term tube feeding. However, a notable disadvantage includes physical extension up to 10 inches outside of the body, increasing the risk of accidental self-removal by the patient via pulling on the tubing. Like G tubes, PEGs also have a risk of local inflammation, dislocation, aspiration, and faults/obstruction of the tube (Table 4.2).

TABLE 4.2 Continuous vs. bolus feeding

Feeding method	Advantages	Disadvantages	Indications
Continuous	• May improve tolerance • May reduce risk of aspiration • Increased time for nutrient absorption	• Feeding pump required • May restrict ambulation • More expensive	• Initiation of feeding in critically ill patients • Promote tolerance • Compromised gastric function Feeding into small bowel Intolerance to other feeding methods
Bolus *Only given through NG/G tubes (bolus feeds *should not* be given for post-pyloric feeding, i.e., ND or NJ tubes)	• More physiological • Feeding pump not required • Inexpensive and easy administration • Limits feeding time • Patient is free to move about, participate in rehabilitation therapies, and live a relatively normal life	• Increased risk of aspiration • Hypertonic, high-fat, or high-fiber formulas may delay gastric emptying or result in osmotic diarrhea	• Recommended for gastric feeding • Normal gastric function

Table adapted from Ichimaru S. Methods of Enteral Nutrition Administration in Critically Ill Patients: Continuous, Cyclic, Intermittent, and Bolus Feeding. Nutr Clin Pract. 2018 Dec;33 (6):790–795. doi: 10.1002/ncp.10105. Epub 2018 Jun 20. PMID: 29924423

Case Example

A 4-week-old, former 34-week gestational age (38-week corrected gestational age) infant male who was recently discharged from the NICU after a 1-month hospital stay for feeding and growing presents to your outpatient primary care clinic for establishment of care and weight evaluation since discharge. The patient is exclusively formula feeding. Per the patient's mother, the patient has been feeding well and remains on Neosure 24 kcal/oz., consuming 2.5 ounces every 2 h. The mother reports that the patient was started on Neosure 24 kcal/oz. during his NICU admission, and has been maintained on it since discharge. On examination, the patient was determined to have a 35 g/day weight gain since discharge. The patient has subcutaneous fat on the face, extremities, and buttock. The child is under no apparent stress and the remainder of the physical exam is within normal limits.

Case Resolution

Mother was instructed to reduce formula concentration from 24 kcal/oz. to 20 kcal/ounce, as catch-up has been obtained. It was determined that the patient was consuming 150 kcal/kg/day (recall that 110–130 kcal/kg/day is a reasonable estimate for daily requirements).

Case Example

A 1-h-old, former full-term infant female is born via normal spontaneous vaginal delivery. At the time of delivery, meconium stained amniotic fluid was noticed. Bulb suction was provided; however, the infant was quickly noticed to have increased work of breathing and grunting. The NICU team was called to bedside for evaluation and the patient was ultimately transferred to the NICU for respiratory support via CPAP administration. Given the CPAP settings, the patient was kept NPO (nothing by mouth) and started on maintenance IV fluids. Over the course of the next 48 h, the patient remained with persistent elevated respiratory support.

Case Resolution

Due to the risk of liquid aspiration in the setting of CPAP use in conjunction with the prolonged time for which the patient was without oral caloric intake, use of an NG tube for feeding (breastmilk and/or formula) administration became an advantageous option. As the patient had an otherwise functional GI tract, the decision was made to place an NG tube to provide adequate oral caloric intake/short-term nutritional support while patient remained NPO on CPAP.

References

1. Hargrove JL. Does the history of food energy units suggest a solution to "Calorie confusion"? Nutr J. 2007;6:44. https://doi.org/10.1186/1475-2891-6-44.

2. "calorie." Merriam-Webster.com. 2011. https://www.merriam-webster.com (6 March 2022).

3. Larson-Nath C, Biank VF. Clinical review of failure to thrive in pediatric patients. Pediatr Ann. 2016;45(2):e46–9. https://doi.org/10.3928/00904481-20160114-01.

4. The National Academies of Sciences, Engineering, and Medicine. Summary report of the dietary reference intakes 1998.

5. Paul IM, Schaefer EW, Miller JR, et al. Weight change nomograms for the first month after birth. Pediatrics. 2016;138(6):e20162625. https://doi.org/10.1542/peds.2016-2625.

6. Crossland DS, Richmond S, Hudson M, Smith K, Abu-Harb M. Weight change in the term baby in the first 2 weeks of life. Acta Paediatr. 2008;97(4):425–9. https://doi.org/10.1111/j.1651-2227.2008.00685.x.

7. Wright CM, Parkinson KN. Postnatal weight loss in term infants: what is normal and do growth charts allow for it? Arch Dis Child Fetal Neonatal Ed. 2004;89(3):F254–7. https://doi.org/10.1136/adc.2003.026906.

8. Macdonald PD, Ross SR, Grant L, Young D. Neonatal weight loss in breast and formula fed infants. Arch Dis Child Fetal Neonatal Ed. 2003;88(6):F472–6. https://doi.org/10.1136/fn.88.6.f472.

9. Grummer-Strawn LM, Reinold C, Krebs NF. Use of World Health Organization and CDC growth charts for children

aged 0–59 months in the United States. MMWR Recomm Rep. 2010;59(Rr-9):1–15.

10. Zemel BS, Pipan M, Stallings VA, et al. Growth charts for children with down syndrome in the United States. Pediatrics. 2015;136(5):e1204–11. https://doi.org/10.1542/peds.2015-1652.

11. Samour PQ, King K. Pediatric nutrition. 4th ed. Sudbury: Jones & Bartlett; 2011.

12. Koletzko B, Goulet O, Hunt J, Krohn K, Shamir R. 1. Guidelines on Paediatric Parenteral Nutrition of the European Society of Paediatric Gastroenterology, Hepatology and Nutrition (ESPGHAN) and the European Society for Clinical Nutrition and Metabolism (ESPEN), Supported by the European Society of Paediatric Research (ESPR). J Pediatr Gastroenterol Nutr. 2005;41(Suppl 2):S1–87. https://doi.org/10.1097/01.mpg.0000181841.07090.f4.

13. Miyasaka EA, Brown PI, Kadoura S, Harris MB, Teitelbaum DH. The adolescent child with short bowel syndrome: new onset of failure to thrive and need for increased nutritional supplementation. J Pediatr Surg. 2010;45(6):1280–6. https://doi.org/10.1016/j.jpedsurg.2010.02.100.

14. Haliburton B, Mouzaki M, Chiang M, et al. Long-term nutritional morbidity for congenital diaphragmatic hernia survivors: failure to thrive extends well into childhood and adolescence. J Pediatr Surg. 2015;50(5):734–8. https://doi.org/10.1016/j.jpedsurg.2015.02.026.

15. Prince A, Groh-Wargo S. Nutrition management for the promotion of growth in very low birth weight premature infants. Nutr Clin Pract. 2013;28(6):659–68. https://doi.org/10.1177/0884533613506752.

16. Valentine CJ, Fernandez S, Rogers LK, et al. Early amino-acid administration improves preterm infant weight. J Perinatol. 2009;29(6):428–32. https://doi.org/10.1038/jp.2009.51.

17. Lambe C, Poisson C, Talbotec C, Goulet O. Strategies to reduce catheter-related bloodstream infections in pediatric patients receiving home parenteral nutrition: the efficacy of taurolidine-citrate prophylactic-locking. JPEN J Parenter Enteral Nutr. 2018;42(6):1017–25. https://doi.org/10.1002/jpen.1043.

18. Chesney CR. The maintenance need for water in parenteral fluid therapy, by Malcolm A. Holliday, MD, and William E. Segar, MD, Pediatrics, 1957;19:823–832. Pediatrics. 1998;102(1 Pt 2):229–30.

19. Jasani B, Rao S, Patole S. Withholding feeds and transfusion-associated necrotizing enterocolitis in preterm infants: a systematic review. Adv Nutr. 2017;8(5):764–9. https://doi.org/10.3945/an.117.015818.

20. Patel RM, Knezevic A, Shenvi N, et al. Association of red blood cell transfusion, anemia, and necrotizing enterocolitis in very low-birth-weight infants. JAMA. 2016;315(9):889–97. https://doi.org/10.1001/jama.2016.1204.

21. Nützenadel W. Failure to thrive in childhood. Dtsch Arztebl Int. 2011;108(38):642–9. https://doi.org/10.3238/arztebl.2011.0642.

22. Michałowska J. EER calculator—estimated energy requirement. https://www.omnicalculator.com/health/eer-estimated-energy-requirement

23. Henry CJ. Basal metabolic rate studies in humans: measurement and development of new equations. Public Health Nutr. 2005;8(7A):1133–52. https://doi.org/10.1079/phn2005801.

24. Carpenter A, Pencharz P, Mouzaki M. Accurate estimation of energy requirements of young patients. J Pediatr Gastroenterol Nutr. 2015;60(1):4–10. https://doi.org/10.1097/MPG.0000000000000572.

25. Afzal NA, Addai S, Fagbemi A, Murch S, Thomson M, Heuschkel R. Refeeding syndrome with enteral nutrition in children: a case report, literature review and clinical guidelines. Clin Nutr. 2002;21(6):515–20. https://doi.org/10.1054/clnu.2002.0586.

26. Stanga Z, Brunner A, Leuenberger M, et al. Nutrition in clinical practice-the refeeding syndrome: illustrative cases and guidelines for prevention and treatment. Eur J Clin Nutr. 2008;62(6):687–94. https://doi.org/10.1038/sj.ejcn.1602854.

27. Gottrand F, Sullivan PB. Gastrostomy tube feeding: when to start, what to feed and how to stop. Eur J Clin Nutr. 2010;64(1):S17–21. https://doi.org/10.1038/ejcn.2010.43.

28. Crawley-Coha T. A practical guide for the management of pediatric gastrostomy tubes based on 14 years of experience. J Wound Ostomy Continence Nurs. 2004;31(4):193–200. https://doi.org/10.1097/00152192-200407000-00007.

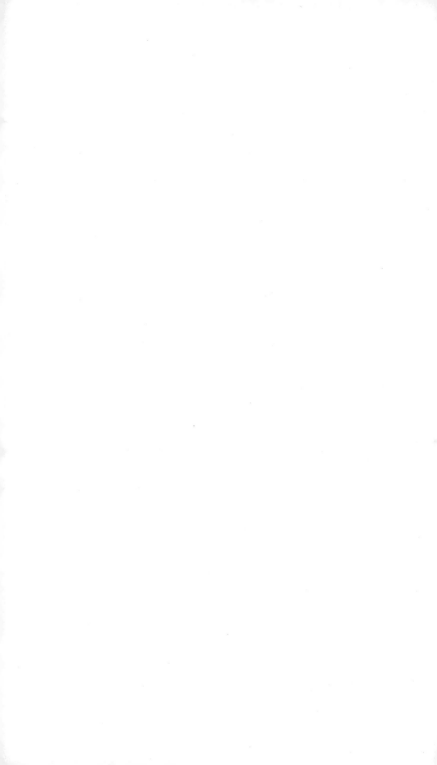

Chapter 5
Management Approach: The Continuum of Care

Gerd McGwire, Allison Heacock, and Tatyana Karakay

Introduction

Failure to thrive (FTT) or faltering growth can present as weight loss, failure to gain weight, or suboptimal growth, with the etiology often being multifactorial and related to the age of the child. Consensus statements and evidence-based recommendations for pediatric malnutrition management exist [1, 2] but there is no comprehensive guideline and few quality studies to specifically guide providers regarding the best management approach for FTT. The care of a child with FTT is often managed in the outpatient setting but it remains a common reason for hospital admission for children less than 24 months of age [3, 4].

G. McGwire (✉) · A. Heacock
Section of Hospital Pediatrics, Nationwide Children's Hospital and The Ohio State University, Columbus, OH, USA
e-mail: Gerd.McGwire@nationwidechildrens.org; Allison.Heacock@nationwidechildrens.org

T. Karakay
Division of Primary Care Pediatrics, Nationwide Children's Hospital and The Ohio State University, Columbus, OH, USA
e-mail: Tatyana.Karakay@nationwidechildrens.org

© Springer Nature Switzerland AG 2023   89
J. G. Vachani (ed.), *Failure to Thrive and Malnutrition*,
https://doi.org/10.1007/978-3-031-14164-5_5

Case Study[1]

A 13-month-old boy presents to the PCP for a delayed 12-month well-child visit. It is noted that the child's rate of weight gain is less than expected. His weight-for-age started flattening at 5 months of age and he is now below the 3rd percentile on the growth chart. The patient presents with his mother and a family friend who provided car transportation to the clinic and who was also asked to help with translation as the mother only speaks Nepali. The medical history is obtained from the mother via an online interpretation service as well as via a family friend. The mother reports that the child eats a traditional, home cooked Nepalese diet. He eats well most of the time but seems to cough a lot during meals and "gets full" quickly. He seems to have less energy than his 4-year-old sister had at his age. On physical exam he appears very anxious. He starts crying and grabs on to his mother as soon as the pediatrician gets close. There are no obvious abnormal exam findings except very scant subcutaneous adipose tissue and maybe a very slight yellowing of the skin, but the exam is significantly limited by the boy's anxiety. The provider ponders what management approach to take to further evaluate and treat this child's failure to thrive.

Management Approach

General Concepts

A patient-centered management approach that is evidence-based and efficient is necessary to achieve high-quality care [5]. Coordination of care is desired in terms of communication as well as physical location, for example, by the establishment of one-stop-shop multidisciplinary clinics [6–8]. Social

---

[1] Although the story in this Case Study is based off actual work performed by a team at Nationwide Children's Hospital, Columbus, Ohio, the patient is fictitious and any resemblance to actual persons, living or dead, is purely coincidental

determinants of health (SDOH) assessment should be included when determining the likely cause of the FTT as well as to identify barriers to the best possible patient outcome. The management approach must be equitable and attentive to cultural preferences of the family.

Multifactorial Diagnosis

Diagnostic evaluation and treatment of a child presenting to an outpatient clinic with FTT can be challenging for a variety of reasons. The heterogeneity of the FTT population makes it difficult to develop and apply an algorithmic, standardized evaluation and management process. A nutrition assessment and examination of length/height in addition to weight parameters is a critical first step to determine whether the infant or child with FTT has malnutrition with or without stunting. Documentation of malnutrition severity is important to justify the need for higher level care as well as for reimbursement purposes. When insufficient caloric intake is suspected—psychosocial, behavioral, and environmental causes are common. In many situations, the history can provide enough information to identify the reason for a child's poor weight gain and allow for effective intervention to improve outcomes. For example, when parents mix formula incorrectly or do not provide adequate amounts of properly prepared formula due to a simple misunderstanding, clear instructions and teaching can completely change the trajectory of a child's outcome. Parents who report having a "happy and content" baby with FTT could suggest that the infant does not communicate hunger cues, like crying, effectively and may thus be left to sleep through the night prematurely. Setting up a more appropriate feeding schedule could then be sufficient to resolve the FTT. Gathering objective information about types and quantities of food the child consumes or the way formula and food are prepared is important as well as a thorough review of systems to identify intolerance of feeds or symptoms that would point to a medical/organic nature of weight gain problems. In some situations, the history and exam can fail to identify any problems and questions about etiology remain unanswered. Communication problems and knowledge gaps—such as a lack of firsthand knowledge by a parent or guardian who is not the primary caregiver, multiple caregivers with insufficient intercommunication, language barrier, and poor recall—can also affect the quality of the information received.

A comprehensive investigation often requires additional steps and strategies to gathering objective, reliable data [9–11]. Examples of such steps include observation of a feeding or a meal and observation of parent–child interaction. An illness-related etiology, such as a neurologic or genetic condition, also needs to be considered during the initial diagnostic evaluation [3, 4, 12–15]. While evidence shows that only around 1–3% of laboratory tests and imaging are of assistance in elucidating a cause of the FTT, the PCP needs to determine if laboratory evaluation is warranted based on history, abnormal physical exam findings, and severity of malnutrition. For example, an upper GI study or head CT might be indicated in a child with FTT and vomiting, the presence of dysmorphic features may lead a practitioner to consider genetic testing and referral to genetics and subspecialty clinics, and increased exertion with feeds may require cardiology workup or referral. The majority of patients, however, will likely not benefit from laboratory testing, imaging, or other diagnostic studies [3, 4, 14–16]. In these instances, a multidisciplinary team evaluation to gather objective data may be the next step in the diagnostic approach.

Pearls

- A comprehensive FTT evaluation requires a nutritional assessment and a detailed history of behavioral, environmental, and psychosocial factors impacting nutrition intake.
- Laboratory testing and imaging are usually of low value and unlikely to lead to a diagnosis.

Multidisciplinary Management

A multidisciplinary approach to evaluation and management of a patient with failure to thrive has been proven to be effective [17–20]. Who should be on the multidisciplinary FTT team?

In outpatient clinics teams typically consist of PCPs and nursing. When available, support from a social worker or psychologist provides valuable information about aspects of a family's life and SDOH including food or housing insecurity, unstable or high-risk living situation, and challenges with parental coping. Certified lactation counselor availability significantly expedites time for mother and infant to get help with any breastfeeding concerns. For formula-fed infants and older children, interventions such as feeding behavior modifications, concentrating formula, the addition of 30 kcal/oz. drink supplements, or adding fats to solid foods can be tried. A study showed that patients in a gastroenterology clinic all gained weight when adherent to such interventions [14]. A registered dietitian and/or occupational therapist may be necessary to help set up and implement these interventions. Providers in outpatient practices may not have access to multidisciplinary professionals easily available, which limits the evaluation and therapies that can be performed in a timely manner. In these cases, referrals such as those to a pediatric gastroenterologist may be needed. The access to affiliated healthcare professionals and subspecialists can be limited depending on the community and the time required to arrange for such referrals. This might lead the PCP to wait until additional interventions, appropriate for age and degree of malnutrition have been attempted and their success evaluated [14].

Pearls

- Due to the multifactorial causation of FTT, a multi- and interdisciplinary team with expertise in all areas of pediatric feeding and growth is key to successful patient outcomes.

- A SW evaluation is highly suggested for all patients admitted for FTT and a full psychosocial assessment should be performed.

If hospitalization is required, pediatric hospitalists and care coordination/case management are added to the team. In addition, hospital-based registered dieticians, social workers, occupational/speech therapists, lactation consultants, and additional subspecialists such as gastroenterologists are often included to aid in a comprehensive, multidisciplinary diagnostic evaluation and construction of an evidence-based treatment plan.

Multidisciplinary teamwork requires clear communication, which can be facilitated by standardized templates for outpatient notes as well as an admission FTT History & Physical Exam (H&P) note. These templates can serve as a clinical support tool for care providers to document important information—such as whether the intent of the primary care provider was to admit due to inadequate response to specific outpatient interventions or to assess the interaction between child and caregiver—as well as provide a standardized format for the inclusion of anthropometric data and designation of malnutrition severity. While the designation of organic versus inorganic FTT is often considered inadequate due to its multifactorial nature, child protective services may require this documentation when involved in a patient's care [12, 13]. Institutions should tailor such communication to the standards of practice in their local environment.

Finally, parents/guardians may request to include key members of their social support system on the team. A patient-centered atmosphere is helpful to help identify each family's process for medical decision-making, implementation, and sustainability of recommended therapies.

The Continuum of Care

The Outpatient Perspective

As discussed above, the extent of the diagnostic evaluation and implementation of therapies for a child with FTT in outpatient clinics have limitations. The biggest hindrance to any FTT investigation or intervention in the outpatient primary care clinic may be time. The evaluation is usually limited to gathering information via the caregiver interview and short observations of the family dynamics during visits. To reliably identify problems related to parent–child interaction, a more prolonged observation period is often required than the usual 15 min allocated for routine visits. When the time or level of care required is not feasible or appropriate in the outpatient setting, admission to the hospital may be the best next step in the management.

Examples of scenarios where admission may be considered include:

- Patients with severe malnutrition.
- Concern for a serious underlying medical condition that necessitates inpatient monitoring and management.
- When inpatient-level evaluation of psychosocial interaction between child and caregiver is deemed necessary.
- When there is a need for precise documentation of nutritional intake.
- Failed outpatient management (i.e., available and recommended outpatient management strategies have been attempted and the child continues to fail to gain adequate weight).

Options can include direct admission to an inpatient unit or a referral to the ED for initial evaluation. Unless the patient exhibits signs of medical instability, including dehydration, electrolyte abnormality, hypothermia, bradycardia, hypotension, or other complications, direct admission if available is usually recommended as this process is perceived to have higher patient satisfaction, reduced risk of nosocomial infection, earlier patient access to pediatric-specific care in hospitals that lack pediatric EDs, and decreased health care costs [21, 22]. Any concern for abuse should trigger a referral for immediate evaluation in the ED. If available, primary care SW should be involved in direct communication of concerns to ED and inpatient SWs to ensure continuity of care. For a direct admission to occur, a system needs to be in place to verify that patient meets the accepting institutions' direct admission requirements and for effective handoff between referring and accepting healthcare providers.

The Inpatient Perspective

From the inpatient provider's perspective, availability of all the information gathered by the PCP as well as the results of the outpatient evaluation and treatment plan is paramount to establish an effective plan of care for the admission. If the PCP has a long-standing relationship with the family or even a detailed patient history for a single visit, this adds additional context to the objective data gathered by the inpatient team at the time of admission. Ideally, inpatient providers and PCPs can view patient medical record information via electronic health record (EHR) data sharing portals to fully comprehend the patient and family dynamic and optimize the continuum of care. A verbal communication between the outpatient and inpatient provider is desired to convey this information as well as to align management plans and goals. Similar information will be obtained from parents/guardians at the time of admission and having the two different perspectives are often necessary to get a complete view of the situation.

Sharing of Information

In addition to the history, the inpatient team relies on the PCP to obtain longitudinal data on growth failure and progression, including details on heights, weights, and head circumferences over time. This information is necessary to determine if the patient has malnutrition and if so, to what extent [2]. If the PCP has any concerns regarding the child's physical exam, this should be shared. Any concerns for neglect/abuse should be reported directly to child protective services (CPS) and communicated between providers at care transitions. If the PCP had the family complete a feeding log, this can provide continuity of care and aid the diagnostic process [9]. The PCP may have additional insights about the parent–child interaction over time, such as cultural customs and diet preferences. Information about family composition and parenting styles can be very helpful to customize the inpatient plan to best fit the child as well as the family. SDOH such as food insecurity, lack of access to reliable transportation, inadequate housing, and a lack of high-quality childcare is a common cause or contributor to FTT and may not always be reported to the inpatient team by the child's caregiver. The PCP might recognize low health literacy or difficulty with adherence to care plans. When SDOH information and barriers to the outpatient FTT management plan are communicated to the inpatient team, the implementation of the inpatient plan can be customized to ensure effectiveness even after discharge.

Aligning Provider Expectations

Effective collaboration and sharing of information between the outpatient and inpatient teams is vital to the success of a child's long-term outcome. Having a comprehensive guideline or clinical pathway that outlines outpatient and inpatient management as well as criteria and process for transitions of care helps set appropriate expectations and achieve high quality and value of care across the continuum [23]. Communication and transparency about reason for admission as well as alignment of goals of the admission are important in order to provide continuity of care for patients and their families and facilitate shared decision-making. Unless there are signs or symptoms suspicious of a medical condition, the inpatient diagnostic evaluation usually starts and may end with a feeding evaluation and monitoring of the parent's and child's proficiency and response to an appropriate feeding regimen. Diagnostic testing indicated by the outpatient evaluation or recommended by the outpatient provider should be communicated at the time of admission so they can be completed or addressed prior to discharge without the need for repeat visits.

While there is a lack of evidence on specific FTT discharge criteria, certain conditions are important and should be met. This includes medical stability including normal mental status, normal or acceptable diagnostic tests, appropriate fluid and caloric intake, stable or increasing weight, and appropriate patient–caregiver interaction prior to discharge. In addition, necessary education must be complete and caregivers must fully understand the discharge and follow-up plan. Whenever possible follow-up by the PCP should be scheduled prior to discharge.

Pearls

- A close cooperation between inpatient and outpatient providers is beneficial to verify the need for an FTT admission, adherence to discharge plan, and successful long-term patient outcome.

Case Study Update[1]

The 13-month-old boy with poor weight gain since 5 months of age was admitted to the Pediatric Hospital Medicine service on the hospital's FTT clinical pathway for further diagnostic evaluation and treatment. A feeding evaluation by the speech pathologist and feeding psychologist revealed an oral aversion, which the parents had previously interpreted as satiety. A nutrition consult developed a feeding plan with table foods, calorie count, and supplementary high caloric nutrition drinks. Targeted lab tests were sent for evaluation of mild icterus and revealed a low level of serum ceruloplasmin potentially concerning for Wilson disease. The family was referred to a comprehensive feeding clinic where a longitudinal management plan was initiated to support the family's feeding dynamic.

Hospital Discharge Communication

The discharge summary has traditionally been the cornerstone of communication from the inpatient team to the pediatric patient's PCP. Discharge summary failures have been shown to lead to patient harm [24, 25]. Therefore, it is important for this document to be timely, accurate, and complete. Several articles have described elements that should be included in a pediatric discharge summary. These include dates of admission and discharge, a brief hospital course, a discharge medication list, a list of follow-up appointments, pending lab or test results, and any immunizations given [26, 27]. These rules should be applied to a patient discharged after admission for FTT. A hospital course including observations of parent–child interaction, feeding technique/schedule, details from a psychosocial assessment, information from consultant evaluation, and a discharge diagnosis (FTT etiology) should also be considered. Documented weight gain during admission might be desired in patients with severe FTT to ensure medical stability and adequate correction of any associated electrolyte or metabolic derangements. Providing the PCP with the instructions parents were given in the hospital, including what patient is supposed to eat and drink (how much, how often, how prepared) with any specific instructions from specialists (including speech therapist, occupational therapist, or dietitian) allows the PCP to reinforce what parents were taught and continue building on that success. The discharge summary should allow the PCP to understand exactly what parents are supposed to do after discharge so any discrepancies can be easily noted and addressed at the follow-up visit.

References

1. Mehta NM, Corkins MR, Lyman B, Malone A, Goday PS, Carney LN, et al. Defining pediatric malnutrition: a paradigm shift toward etiology-related definitions. JPEN J Parenter Enteral Nutr. 2013;37(4):460–81.
2. Bouma S. Diagnosing pediatric malnutrition: paradigm shifts of etiology-related definitions and appraisal of the indicators. Nutr Clin Pract. 2017;32(1):52–67.
3. Larson-Nath C, St Clair N, Goday P. Hospitalization for failure to thrive: a prospective descriptive report. Clin Pediatr (Phila). 2018;57(2):212–9.
4. Sills RH. Failure to thrive. The role of clinical and laboratory evaluation. Am J Dis Child. 1978;132(10):967–9.
5. Institute of Medicine Committee on Quality of Health Care in America. Crossing the quality chasm: a new health system for the 21st century. Washington, DC: National Academies Press (US); 2001. Copyright 2001 by the National Academy of Sciences. All rights reserved
6. Knight RM, Albright JJ, Huth-Bocks A, Morris NK, Mills L, Klok K, et al. Impact of behavioral feeding intervention on child emotional and behavioral functioning, parenting stress, and parent-child attachment. J Pediatr Gastroenterol Nutr. 2019;69(3):383–7.
7. Jung JS, Chang HJ, Kwon JY. Overall profile of a pediatric multidisciplinary feeding clinic. Ann Rehabil Med. 2016;40(4):692–701.
8. Luscombe GM, Hawthorn J, Wu A, Green B, Munro A. 'Empowering clinicians in smaller sites': a qualitative study of clinician's experiences with a rural virtual paediatric feeding clinic. Aust J Rural Health. 2021;29(5):742–52.
9. Lezo A, Baldini L, Asteggiano M. Failure to thrive in the outpatient clinic: a new insight. Nutrients. 2020;12(8):2202.
10. Homan GJ. Failure to thrive: a practical guide. Am Fam Physician. 2016;94(4):295–9.
11. Faltering growth: recognition and management of faltering growth in children [Internet]. 2017. Available from https://www.nice.org.uk/guidance/ng75/chapter/Recommendations
12. Jaffe AC. Failure to thrive: current clinical concepts. Pediatr Rev. 2011;32(3):100–7. quiz 8

13. Larson-Nath C, Biank VF. Clinical review of failure to thrive in pediatric patients. Pediatr Ann. 2016;45(2):e46–9.
14. Larson-Nath CM, Goday PS. Failure to thrive: a prospective study in a pediatric gastroenterology clinic. J Pediatr Gastroenterol Nutr. 2016;62(6):907–13.
15. Selbuz S, Kırsaçlıoğlu CT, Kuloğlu Z, Yılmaz M, Penezoğlu N, Sayıcı U, et al. Diagnostic workup and micronutrient deficiencies in children with failure to thrive without underlying diseases. Nutr Clin Pract. 2019;34(4):581–8.
16. Berwick DM, Levy JC, Kleinerman R. Failure to thrive: diagnostic yield of hospitalisation. Arch Dis Child. 1982;57(5):347–51.
17. Wright CM, Callum J, Birks E, Jarvis S. Effect of community based management in failure to thrive: randomised controlled trial. BMJ. 1998;317(7158):571–4.
18. Hobbs C, Hanks HG. A multidisciplinary approach for the treatment of children with failure to thrive. Child Care Health Dev. 1996;22(4):273–84.
19. Bithoney WG, McJunkin J, Michalek J, Snyder J, Egan H, Epstein D. The effect of a multidisciplinary team approach on weight gain in nonorganic failure-to-thrive children. J Dev Behav Pediatr. 1991;12(4):254–8.
20. Atalay A, McCord M. Characteristics of failure to thrive in a referral population: implications for treatment. Clin Pediatr (Phila). 2012;51(3):219–25.
21. Leyenaar JK, Shieh MS, Lagu T, Pekow PS, Lindenauer PK. Direct admission to hospitals among children in the United States. JAMA Pediatr. 2015;169(5):500–2.
22. Leyenaar JK, O'Brien ER, Malkani N, Lagu T, Lindenauer PK. Direct admission to hospital: a mixed methods survey of pediatric practices, benefits, and challenges. Acad Pediatr. 2016;16(2):175–82.
23. Lion KC, Wright DR, Spencer S, Zhou C, Del Beccaro M, Mangione-Smith R. Standardized clinical pathways for hospitalized children and outcomes. Pediatrics. 2016;137(4):e20151202.
24. Gattari TB, Krieger LN, Hu HM, Mychaliska KP. Medication discrepancies at pediatric hospital discharge. Hosp Pediatr. 2015;5(8):439–45.
25. Larrow A, Chong A, Robison T, Patel A, Kuelbs C, Fisher E, et al. A quality improvement initiative to improve discharge timeliness and documentation. Pediatr Qual Saf. 2021;6(4):e440.

26. Leyenaar JK, Desai AD, Burkhart Q, Parast L, Roth CP, McGalliard J, et al. Quality measures to assess care transitions for hospitalized children. Pediatrics. 2016;138(2):e20160906.
27. Coghlin DT, Leyenaar JK, Shen M, Bergert L, Engel R, Hershey D, et al. Pediatric discharge content: a multisite assessment of physician preferences and experiences. Hosp Pediatr. 2014;4(1):9–15.

Chapter 6
Failure to Thrive and Population Health: The Impact of Disparities and Social Determinants

Deborah A. Frank and Steven Rogers

Introduction: Failure to Thrive (FTT), also termed in recent publications as growth faltering, has been historically categorized as either organic—arising from major organ dysfunction or a congenital/genetic disease—or non-organic—not stemming from one of these conditions but instead an indicator of "environmental deprivation." For ease of comparison with decades of medical/psychological literature, in this chapter we will continue to use the traditional label "Failure to Thrive (FTT)", while acknowledging that it is outdated. More recent evidence suggests that there are typically several factors at play in each case of FTT, demonstrating that the organic/nonorganic dichotomy is overly simplistic [1]. The organic/nonorganic distinction was also problematic because nonorganic FTT was often ascribed to the individual failure of mothers to nurture infants adequately, typically as a result of their own psychological deficits [2, 3]. This placed undue blame on families, particularly mothers, who may not have

D. A. Frank (✉) · S. Rogers
Department of Pediatrics, Boston University School of Medicine, Boston Medical Center, Boston, MA, USA

Children's Hospital of Philadelphia, Philadelphia, PA, USA
e-mail: dafrank@bu.edu; srrogers@bu.edu

© Springer Nature Switzerland AG 2023
J. G. Vachani (ed.), *Failure to Thrive and Malnutrition*,
https://doi.org/10.1007/978-3-031-14164-5_6

had the resources to provide adequate nutrition for their children, regardless of their intentions or psychological state.

Poverty is a major predictor of FTT. Social circumstances make major contributions to the overall risk of this condition, regardless of whether other medical factors are also present. These circumstances fall under the broader rubric of social determinants of health (SDH): the conditions in which people are born, live, grow, and age [4]. These social determinants of health include food insecurity, housing instability, energy insecurity, and lack of adequate childcare. SDH should be identified and whenever possible addressed with the same rigor as potential predisposing medical and developmental conditions. Health care access and affordability are an SDH that is beyond the scope of this chapter.

Social determinants of health influence the potential trajectory of a child's growth beginning with the mother's nutrition and health status even before conception. As pregnancy proceeds, these factors help determine the birth weight and other indicators of perinatal health [5]. Prematurity, low birth weight, and other perinatal conditions increase subsequent risk of poor weight gain and FTT [6, 7]. This chapter will discuss the role of SDH in FTT along with the management of FTT in multidisciplinary care models, which when combined with other interventions seek to mitigate the impact of these SDH on children's growth and development.

Failure to Thrive and Population Health

Birth weight and postnatal childhood weight-for-age, stunting, and body mass index are classic indicators of population health throughout the developed and developing world as readily measured indicators of developmental potential, risk of excess morbidity and mortality in infancy and early childhood, and predictive factors of later adult health and premature mortality [8–10]. Because the rate of low birth weight is higher than the infant mortality rate across the United States, low birth weight can be a more reliable measure than infant mortality rate for smaller sample sizes and when studying regions with smaller populations [11, 12].

Low birth weight has been shown to be a predictor of future FTT in children, with those born at very low birth weight (VLBW, <1500 g) at increased risk for future growth deficiencies compared to those born over 1500 g [6, 13, 14]. Infants with birth weight < 2500 g have a risk of growth failure of 19.7%, a risk which increases to 28% for the subset of these infants born <1000 g [6, 7]. The risk of adverse cognitive outcomes is higher in children with both low birth weight and subsequent FTT than with either condition alone; it is therefore of great importance that low birth weight children are monitored closely for subsequent faltering in growth and they receive interventions as soon as growth faltering is identified [6].

The relative impact of risk factors for FTT differs based on the population being studied. In low-income countries low birth weight, recurrent infectious diseases, extreme poverty, and inconsistent access to adequate medical care and nutrition represent the major risks to children's growth [15]. In high-income countries these factors also play a role but low birth weight—whether attributable to prematurity or intrauterine growth retardation—and family dysfunction and adverse social determinants may be more potent [15].

Social Determinants of Health and FTT

Social determinants of health—the conditions in which people are born, grow, live, work, and age—are particularly salient in the diagnosis and management of failure to thrive [16]. The immediate causes of FTT are now understood to be multifactorial, with contributions made by physical illnesses, social factors, nutrition, and disorders of development [17]. Of the social contributors to FTT, the most significant upstream risk factor is poverty [17]. The harmful effects of poverty on child health are by no means limited to weight status. Compared to those living in higher-income families, children in low-income families have an increased risk of medical conditions such as asthma as well as behavioral issues linked to several dimensions of poverty including low income, material deprivation, and subjective financial stress [18, 19]. A study utilizing data from the 2009 Pediatric Nutrition Surveillance Study found that 6% of children between birth and 4 years of age who qualified for federal nutrition assistance because of low family income were of short stature, compared to 3.7% of all US children of the same age [20]. The mechanism by which poverty increases risk of FTT is through its association with more proximate social determinants of health, including food insecurity, energy insecurity, and housing instability. In the case of food insecurity, families who are unable to afford more nutrient-rich food are often limited to buying inexpensive, nutrient-poor, energy-dense food. This staves off hunger in the short term but provides insufficient and inconsistent macronutrients and micronutrients for children's normal growth [21].

Food Insecurity

Food insecurity can be further characterized as either low food security (reports of reduced quality, variety, or desirability of diet, with little or no indication of reduced food intake) or very low food security (reports of multiple indications of disrupted eating patterns and reduced food intake). Because of its high prevalence and clear mechanistic link to FTT, food insecurity is perhaps the most significant immediate social determinant of FTT. Food insecurity continues to be a major problem in the United States affecting 10.5% of households according to the USDA estimates for 2020; 11.7 million children lived in these food-insecure households, and 6.1 million children were estimated to personally experience food insecurity [22]. Some children are insulated from the effects of food insecurity at the household level, as some adults will cut back on their own intake before doing so for their children. However, overall rate of food insecurity in households with children was 14.8% in 2020 during the first year of the COVID pandemic rose from 13.6% in 2019. According to data from the Household Pulse Survey, during the Coronavirus Pandemic, the overall trend in food insecurity greatly increased at the onset of the pandemic, followed by a decrease in 2021. Food insecurity does not affect all families equally, as became more apparent during the pandemic. During this time period, low-income families and Black- or Hispanic-headed households were more likely to experience food insecurity than above-low-income households or households with a head identifying as white. Households with children were more likely to report that their households did not get enough to eat than those without children during this period (14% compared to 8%). There remains considerable variation in the prevalence of household food insecurity based on geographic location, ranging from 5.7% of all households in New Hampshire to 15.3% of all households in Mississippi from 2018 to 2020 (USDA) [22].

Though the overall evidence base has not reliably found a specific association between food insecurity and FTT in children at the population level, food insecurity remains a frequent clinical finding among low-income children with FTT [23]. There is some data from the United States indicating that the effect of food insecurity on child weight status is dependent on the timing of exposure, with children experiencing food insecurity in kindergarten having higher risk of underweight in eighth grade, while those experiencing food insecurity later in childhood having higher average BMIs in eighth grade [24].

Food insecurity has also been found to be associated with an increased risk of hospitalization since birth, parent-reported fair/poor health status, asthma and other chronic conditions, and iron deficiency anemia [25–28]. Additionally, food insecurity has a negative effect on the learning and performance of children in school, and on noncognitive skills, which include interpersonal relations and self-control [23, 29]. Finally, food insecurity has been shown to be associated with maternal depression [30]. For many families, food insecurity is a recurrent but not constant condition, dependent on the timing of receipt of paychecks and benefits; food insecurity, therefore, warrants careful and repeated evaluation for this remediable risk factor as children are receiving ongoing care for FTT.

Housing and Physical Environment

Inadequate housing may also be associated with weight status in children. The effects of housing instability and homelessness on child health begin during the prenatal period, as homelessness during pregnancy has been found to be associated with an increased risk of low birth weight and preterm delivery [31, 32]. Lifetime history of homelessness or housing instability (defined based on circumstances including multiple recent moves or being behind on rent or mortgage within the past year) has been found to be associated with an increased risk of several adverse child health outcomes, but not with increased risk of being underweight [33]. Inadequate housing is itself a stressor, but also promotes infectious respiratory and gastrointestinal illnesses through exposure to unsanitary conditions and close contact with ill family members. Inadequate housing can also be viewed as an effect of general financial strain, which reduces discretionary income that can be used to promote child health through healthy food and other means.

One specific mechanism by which unhealthy housing can contribute to FTT is through lead exposure. Studies have shown that lower household income is associated with elevated blood lead levels in children [34–36]. Though overall trends in mean childhood blood levels have been reassuring (CDC), recent high-profile cases including that of Flint, Michigan demonstrate that the potential for lead exposure is still a cause for concern, especially in low-income areas [37]. Childhood malnutrition and FTT may actually increase the risk for lead poisoning in children, as malnourished children are more likely to be anemic secondary to iron deficiency, which increases the absorption of lead through shared iron-lead transporters in the gut [38]. This mechanistic link, along with evidence that children with FTT have been found to have significantly elevated blood lead levels compared to healthy controls, reinforces the importance of screening for blood lead levels, particularly in populations living in at-risk areas [39]. In spite of some controversy about universal screening, screening for children 12–24 months of age in communities with ≥25% of housing built prior to 1960 or a ≥5% prevalence of children's blood lead concentrations ≥5 μg/dL is recommended at every anthropometric level [40].

Energy Insecurity

Energy insecurity, an inability to adequately meet basic energy needs because of cost, is another social determinant of health, which can contribute to FTT in part by a further straining of limited family financial resources [41]. Energy insecurity is particularly problematic for those living in colder climates, where families are sometimes forced to choose between paying energy bills to ensure their homes remain heated or paying for food, in what has been called the "heat or eat" dilemma. There is some related evidence that the percentage of children brought to the emergency department with a weight-for-age below the fifth percentile is higher following the coldest months than the remaining months of the year, and that poor families report reducing their expenditures on food by approximately the same degree that they have to increase their expenditures on energy during cold shocks [42, 43]. Energy insecurity in warmer months and climates can also have deleterious effects on child health. There is evidence that high ambient temperature may be associated with increased risk of sudden infant death syndrome, as well as low birth weight [44, 45]. Energy insecurity like inadequate housing can be viewed as a downstream effect of poverty, which constrains a family's ability to have enough available income to purchase sufficient amounts of food while meeting other basic needs. These forms of material hardship that jeopardize child health are tightly linked as meager resources allocated to one need can leave the others unmet. The family may never be secure in all domains simultaneously. The food budget is often the one most readily diverted to other urgent needs as families appropriately fear immediate homelessness or lack of light and heat but the effects of insufficient food are generally more insidious. Clinicians caring for children with FTT should repeatedly screen for all dimensions of hardship, especially when a child's growth falters without an obvious explanation for acute illness [19, 46].

Caregiver Factors

Poverty can exert a profound effect on children not only through concrete forms of material deprivation summarized above but also through its influence on the socio-emotional functioning of parents and other caregivers. Though the categories of "organic" and "inorganic" FTT are no longer considered optimal for the characterization of this condition, the fact that this fallacious distinction has been able to persist for so many years does highlight the importance of evaluating family and caregiver factors [47].

Major depression is a common condition that is linked to poverty, and one which may profoundly impact the children of affected caregivers. The risk of a major depressive episode has been found to be higher in those of low socioeconomic status, and also in African Americans compared to Whites [48, 49]. Unmet material needs may trigger parental depression. A study of over 5000 mothers found an association between positive depression screens and recently reduced or lost food stamps or other government benefits, household food insecurity, fair or poor child health, and hospitalization of their child since birth; this study did not detect a direct association between maternal depression and child growth [30]. Overall, the evidence base for a direct association between maternal depression and FTT in children is mixed.

There is some evidence that the risk of depression is higher in mothers of children with growth faltering and that chronic maternal depression is associated with reduced weight gain in select populations of infants particularly in developing countries [50–52]. However, the link does not appear to persist in high-resource countries [53–55]. The presence of the potential confounding effects of poverty are often not assessed in studies, which makes it difficult to detect any direct association between maternal depression and FTT. The fact that caring for a child with FTT itself could contribute to caregiver depression further complicates the picture [54]. It may be most helpful to conceptualize caregiver depression as the possible result of any combination of many interpersonal and biologic/genetic factors exacerbated by poverty-related negative SDH (e.g., food insecurity or barriers to sufficient wages or government assistance) and that these same SDH may also contribute directly to FTT in the children of these caregivers. Regardless of whether a direct causal link exists between caregiver depression and FTT, a wholistic approach that involves treating parental distress as well as the child's nutritional and developmental deficits in remediating FTT is warranted.

Child abuse is another caregiver-related factor that can contribute to FTT. A review of prior literature determined that children with FTT were four times more likely than children without FTT to be sexually and/or physically abused, though the overall percentage of children with FTT with reported cases of abuse was low, at 5–10% [56]. Several major risk factors for abuse in a child with suspected FTT are related to SDH, particularly poverty [57]. However, despite the association between child abuse and FTT, it is important that clinicians keep in mind that the vast majority of children with FTT have not been physically or sexually abused. Child abuse should not become a diagnosis by exclusion and should not be conflated with poverty itself [58]. This should also be kept in mind in cases of suspected child neglect, as a situation in which parents are doing their best to care for a child in the setting of extreme poverty might be mistaken for negligence.

Finally, parental dietary beliefs and practices, separate from those that come about as a result of poverty, can also contribute to the development of FTT in children. Examples include parental veganism in exclusively breast-fed infants, which has been implicated in nutrient deficiencies (particularly vitamin B_{12}) and subsequent FTT in case studies [59, 60]. Excessive fruit juice intake, while sometimes viewed as a cause of overweight in children, has also been associated with FTT [61]. While fruit juice may be used in low-income households as a means of achieving satiety in children when other food is not available, excessive juice intake in children (sometimes contributing to diarrhea) may also be the result of uninformed dietary choices made on the part of their parents [62].

Lack of Consensus on the Link Between Poverty and FTT

Though plausible mechanistic links between poverty and FTT have been described, it should be acknowledged that the degree to which the two are directly associated has been challenged [63]. A study of children in the United Kingdom found that the families of children with FTT were similar to controls in markers of poverty, suggesting that the role of poverty in the development of FTT might be overestimated for certain populations [56]. A longitudinal population cohort study, also performed in the United Kingdom, found no association between low weight gain among infants and traditional markers of poverty, but did find an association with parental height and parity [64]. Generalizability of the previously mentioned studies to the United States may be limited, given the United Kingdom's more robust system of child social supports and universal health care access at baseline. Consistent with results from the United Kingdom, a study of hospitalized children in the United States compared those with a diagnosis of malnutrition (which included FTT) with controls and did not find a significant difference in family income between the two groups [65]. Although consensus is lacking on a simple association between income poverty and FTT, logic and experience mandate a careful assessment of income-related stressors, including the SDH enumerated here. Studies of poverty's association with FTT should not just consider income poverty, but multiple dimensions of deprivation which can impact outcomes even if family income is higher than the formal poverty level—including the material hardships noted above and subjective financial stress [19].

The evidence supporting an association between poverty and child malnutrition in general (including obesity) is more robust [66–68]. A lack of nutrition of adequate quality and quantity for the physiologic needs of the child is (except in the cases of rare inborn errors of metabolism) most often a proximate cause of FTT. Therefore, even if the existence of an indisputable association between poverty and FTT itself has not yet been clearly established in all high-resource countries, poverty cannot be ruled out as an upstream risk factor for FTT as it clearly influences the more proximate causes of this condition. One factor potentially obscuring a direct association between poverty and FTT is the more significant effect of long-term poverty compared to short-term poverty on child nutritional status; studies of poverty's effects which rely on cross-sectional data may therefore miss the longitudinal effects of cumulative and persistent poverty on the family function and the children's nutritional status [66]. Additionally, the weight status of children living in poverty may be distributed in a bimodal fashion. If child overweight and obesity are far more common in high-income countries than underweight and FTT, focusing only on differences in average weight between income groups makes an association between poverty and each growth extremely difficult to detect. Other potentially confounding elements include the absence of an agreed-upon definition of FTT, the use of inconsistent markers of poverty in each study, and demographic differences between populations in different regions.

Program Participation and Failure to Thrive

Effects of Program Participation on Weight and Growth in Children

Participation in the Supplemental Nutrition Assistance Program (SNAP, formerly Food Stamps), the Special Supplemental Nutrition Program for Women, Infants, and Children (WIC), and/or school meals programs (National School Lunch Program and School Breakfast Program) has been linked to numerous benefits in children and their parents. Any combination of these three programs has been demonstrated to be associated with lower risk of several nutrition-related health problems, including FTT [69]. However, these programs entail many bureaucratic and logistic barriers to access, and do not reach all children who would benefit from their receipt or even all children who live in income-eligible families.

Specific programs have also been studied separately for their effects on weight gain and growth in children. A review of early studies of WIC's effects on the health of children found that WIC participation was associated with increased growth in both weight and length among infants [70]. Subsequent studies have determined that children unable to receive WIC assistance due to access problems were more likely to be underweight and to lag in height [71]. Other positive effects of WIC are visible far earlier than its mitigating effects on FTT, as WIC participation has been linked to improved perinatal health measures including birth weight. Though there were some concerns that early studies of WIC's effectiveness did not properly account for selection bias, in that mothers who sought out this benefit might be healthier and more motivated than mothers who did not, a study comparing WIC participants to nonparticipant mothers who were automatically eligible by virtue of their Medicaid enrollment status found that WIC's positive effects on perinatal health persisted even when recipients were compared to appropriate controls [72, 73]. Many studies have subsequently demonstrated the positive impact of WIC on birth weight [74–76]. Predictably the loss of WIC benefits at 61 months of age once the child has "aged out" of the program has been found to increase risk of food insecurity, representing a particularly vulnerable period for these children [77].

SNAP receipt has also been shown to have positive effects on birth weight and infant growth. A review of birth certificate data from across the United States found that maternal SNAP receipt during pregnancy was associated with increased birth weight: an effect that was more pronounced among recipients in lower-income counties and for infants at the lower end of the birth weight spectrum [78]. The positive effects of SNAP on child growth extend beyond birth, as a recent study found that young children in SNAP recipient households were less likely to be underweight (<5th percentile weight-for-age) than comparison children in households which did not receive SNAP [79]. SNAP's effects on food insecurity—a potential risk factor for FTT—have also been studied, and there is ample data showing that SNAP recipients are less likely to be food insecure than likely eligible controls by up to 30% according to some estimates [79–81].

Nutrition assistance programs are integrated with child care in the Child and Adult Care Food Program (CACFP), which provides reimbursements to child and adult care providers for meals and snacks served to those in their care [82]. During the 2018 fiscal year, these benefits reached child care centers with a total average daily attendance of 4.7 million children, constituting a total of approximately 1.4 billion free meals [83]. There is some evidence that participation in this program is associated with a reduced risk of underweight status among low-income children, demonstrating the importance of improving access to food for children in settings outside the home [82].

In addition to nutrition programs, providers should be aware of other forms of assistance which can mitigate harmful SDH. The Low Income Home Energy Assistance Program (LIHEAP) provides some assistance with energy costs to low-income families but is not an entitlement (i.e., not automatically available to anyone who meets the income and citizenship requirements). Eligibility criteria vary by state, but eligibility is generally based on income (no state can set income eligibility criteria to <110% of the federal poverty level) or can be granted based on receipt of other benefits [84, 85] LIHEAP benefits have been found to be associated with decreased risk of undernutrition in children living in affected households [86, 87]. LIHEAP is not as well-known as the major nutrition assistance programs but is a useful resource for families in need, particularly those in colder climates.

The programs discussed above address the social determinants of food insecurity and energy insecurity, but they are by no means the only relevant social determinants to FTT or the only programs which exist to address them. Social determinants such as housing instability are relevant to FTT and in many ways more difficult to address quickly in the clinical setting through referrals to resources. While an in-depth discussion of all the assistance programs directed at housing and other social needs is beyond the scope of this chapter, clinicians should be aware of their importance in ameliorating this pervasive social determinant of health; for example, receipt of public housing subsidies has been found to be associated with improved nutritional status in children [87, 88].

Regional Regulations Impacting Nutrition Assistance Programs

The rules and regulations pertaining to nutrition assistance programs often vary by state. It would be beneficial for clinicians to become familiar with these regulations, particularly those pertaining to eligibility criteria, to facilitate referrals for families in need. While eligibility criteria and referral processes are too variable to describe in detail in this chapter, some overarching regulations will be discussed.

The previously mentioned nutrition assistance programs are considered to be means tested but not all are entitlements. WIC income eligibility varies by state but must be below 185% of the federal poverty level throughout the country [89]. The National School Breakfast and Lunch Program traditionally provides reduced prices and free meals to those with income below 185% and 130% of the Federal Poverty Level [90]. In some low-income school districts, all students are considered categorically eligible for free meals; because this determination is based on the percentage of students who are already eligible for SNAP and TANF (Temporary Assistance for Needy Families), any change in policy that affects enrollment in these programs also poses the risk of indirectly reducing access to school meals. SNAP— the largest of the USDA's food assistance programs—has a federal gross monthly income limit of 130% of the federal poverty level, meaning that no state can set an income limit below this point [91, 92]. All states have also adopted "traditional" categorical eligibility, in which families that receive certain other benefits (most commonly TANF) are automatically eligible for SNAP. As of 2017, most states had also adopted "broad-based" categorical eligibility, which makes most low-income families eligible for SNAP through receipt of minimal TANF-funded benefits [93]. Proposals from the USDA in 2019 to limit categorical eligibility have been rescinded since the 2020 elections. The case of SNAP illustrates the complexity of regulations surrounding nutrition assistance programs, as well as the importance of having some understanding of these regulations on the part of clinicians to ensure that the maximum number of eligible families who require food assistance receive referrals. The effectiveness of referrals is facilitated by partnerships between clinicians and professionals with expertise in helping families navigate these complex systems.

Variability in Access

Though SNAP and other government nutrition programs have a positive impact on children with FTT, they do not reach all those who are eligible—with wide variation by year and by state [94]. Rates of access to nutrition assistance programs vary across demographic groups. For example, in Texas, a lack of English proficiency proved to be a barrier to SNAP access [95]. A review of peer-reviewed and gray literature pertaining to SNAP participation rates found that eligible individuals are less likely to participate in SNAP in rural areas, possibly because of a lack of accurate information on eligibility criteria and transportation barriers in reaching sites where applications can be submitted, as well as a higher prevalence of adverse attitudes regarding participation in government assistance programs [96]. Overall, it is clear that difficulties in accessing benefits are common among eligible families, and that perceptions surrounding the receipt of these benefits are varied. Clinicians treating children with FTT should be aware of these factors and be prepared to educate families so that they are better able to receive the resources they need.

Immigration Status

Complicating access to government food programs is a matter of immigration status, both of children and their parents. Though eligibility varies by program, undocumented immigrants are generally ineligible for federal public benefits including SNAP, though their American born children are eligible [97, 98]. The documented noncitizens considered "qualified aliens" may be eligible for SNAP after certain work requirements are met, and qualified alien children are generally eligible for SNAP [99]. Other programs, including WIC and the school meals programs, are less restrictive, and as of 2015 all states had opted to designate every child as eligible for WIC and school meals regardless of immigration status [97, 98].

Beyond formal eligibility, perceptions of the dangers involved in the receipt of public benefits may impact the likelihood that immigrant parents seek them out. In a study of caregivers and their children in several US cities, SNAP participation among immigrant families in the United States for less than 5 years (SNAP eligibility begins at more than 5 years for legally present adults, but US born children are immediately eligible increased from 25.4% in 2007 to 43% by 2017 and dropped abruptly in 34.8% in 2018 [100]. Anecdotal evidence suggests that this drop may be the result of increasing fear of deportation in the face of tightening immigration enforcement and what has been perceived as increased anti-immigrant rhetoric in public discourse [101].

Drops in food program participation, especially if driven by anti-immigration rhetoric and policies, are especially concerning considering the relatively high rates of food insecurity among families with immigrant members in the United States, particularly for immigrant Latinx [102]. There is some data suggesting that specific immigration policies themselves may be associated with increases in food insecurity. One study found that the enactment of a short-lived immigration law which allowed for local law enforcement officers to be deputized for immigration enforcement was associated with a 10% increase in food insecurity among Mexican noncitizen households with children in the United States [103].

Management of FTT from a Social Determinants Perspective

The discussion of social determinants of FTT can be a complex one because of the frequency with which social determinants occur together and in varying combinations. The complexity of this situation underlines the importance of a robust screening and referral system that is capable of detecting a wide range of social risk factors and connecting families with the resources necessary to bring about long-term improvements in child health. This system of screening and resource referrals linked with standard medical care may be best achieved through the model of the multidisciplinary clinic, which will be discussed below.

Social Determinants Screening

Detection of exposure to harmful SDH is best accomplished through screening. Though different screens have been developed for specific SDH, some general principles common to effective SDH screening have been identified. SDH screening should be tailored to the target population in terms of area-specific demographics and developmental stage of individual patients [104]. Ideally, widespread screening should only begin after mechanisms are in place to refer patients to effective resources [104]. The logistics of screening can be flexible depending on the resources of the clinic. Both universal screeners and screeners for specific SDH exist and have been proven effective in detecting social needs [4, 105, 106]. Some of these screens have been validated in languages other than English [104]. Screening can be performed in a face-to-face fashion or using electronic devices, although there is some evidence that parents are more likely to report certain sensitive social issues when electronic devices are used [107].

Universal screeners include the Health-Related Social Needs (HRSN) Screening Tool which was developed by the Centers for Medicare and Medicaid Services as a part of their Accountable Health Communities Model, an initiative that seeks to study the effects of systematic social needs screening on health care expenditures [108, 109]. The screener and its supplemental questions are comprehensive and cover domains including food insecurity, housing instability, transportation issues, utility help needs, interpersonal safety, and financial strain [108]. The Protocol for Responding to and Addressing Patient Assets, Risks, and Experiences (PRAPARE) is a tool developed by the National Association of Community Health Centers, which in addition to the usual social factors of food insecurity and housing instability also assesses refugee status and history of incarceration [110].

Finally, the WE CARE screening tool—which assesses the need for child care, education, employment, food security, household heat, and housing—has been found to increase the odds of parental enrollment in new resources and parental employment and to decrease the odds that families lived in a homeless shelter [4]. With such a variety of universal social needs screeners available, a clinic has the ability to choose which one might best suit its specific patient population.

Screening for food insecurity is particularly important given its relatively high prevalence, and potential for serious adverse effects on children's health and development. An extensive, 18-item survey developed by the USDA, called the US Household Food Security Survey Module, is freely available online (USDA ERS) and serves as the gold standard for food insecurity screening [111]. A brief two-item screen for food insecurity—the "Hunger Vital Sign"—has also been validated, and can readily be used in clinical settings [106]. The two items on this screener are: "Within the past 12 months we worried whether our food would run out before we got money to buy more" and "Within the past 12 months the food we bought just didn't last and we didn't have money to get more"; an affirmative response (i.e., "sometimes true" or "often true") to either question was determined to have a sensitivity of 97% and a specificity of 83% compared to the 18-item scale [106]. This effective two-question screener is recommended by the American Academy of Pediatrics, which has promoted screening for food insecurity [112]. This screen has been shown to be effective both in primary care and in emergency department settings, the latter having a higher percentage of children screening positive for food insecurity [113]. Subspecialty programs, especially those dealing with children with FTT or other nutrition-sensitive conditions should also adopt the Hunger Vital Sign.

Social determinants relevant to failure to thrive, and resources available to address them

Domain	Specific social determinants	Available resources
Material needs	Food insecurity	SNAP, WIC, NSLP, SBP, CACFP, charitable food organizations
	Energy insecurity	LIHEAP
Housing	Housing instability	Federal rental assistance, local shelters, city housing authorities
	Crowding	Federal rental assistance, local shelters, city housing authorities
	Housing exposures (e.g. mold, lead)	State and local health departments
Caregiver factors	Parental depression	SAMHSA to locate behavioral health resources
	Child abuse	State Child Protective Services
	Inadequate childcare	State departments of Education/Early Education
Other	Immigration status	Local pro bono legal services

SNAP Supplemental Nutrition Assistance Program, *WIC* Special Supplemental Nutrition Program for Women, Infants, and Children, *NSLP* National School Lunch Program, *SBP* School Breakfast Program, *CACFP* Child and Adult Care Food Program, *LIHEAP* Low Income Home Energy Assistance Program, *SAMHSA* Substance Abuse and Mental Health Services Administration

Effective Referrals to Necessary Resources

To improve the condition of children with FTT and social needs, the detection of these needs must be followed up with effective referrals to resources. These referrals can be made by any member of the health care team and often fall into the purview of social workers or case managers. The Cambridge Health Alliance's Model of Team-Based Care utilizes social workers for complex care management to connect patients with overlapping medical and social needs with resources [114]. While these complex care management teams are typically focused on older adults, their social needs-conscious model might also be well-suited to children at risk for FTT [114].

A list of resources should be kept readily available and up to date, both on resources within the local community and those administered by the state or national governments [4, 115]. To facilitate the identification of community resources and referral of patients to these resources, a number of online platforms now exist, including Aunt Bertha© (recently rebranded as findhelp©) and CharityTracker© [116, 117]. Many of these platforms are available in a free-to-use version for use by the general public as well as in paid versions, which are designed with additional features for use by health care or other professional organizations [118]. However, the cost of the initial setup and continuing subscription fees may prove prohibitive for small or low-resource clinical organizations [118]. In addition to providing detailed information on a number of these platforms, the Social Interventions Research & Evaluation Network (SIREN) recommends that health care organizations personally engage with the leadership of their community partners as soon as possible, to build fruitful relationships that can better serve their patients [118]. Building relationships with charitable food providers who often also undertake assisting clients in applying for public programs is particularly important. These charitable (or philanthropic) feeding resources are invaluable in emergent situations, but are not sustained interventions to support children's nutritional status in the long term. Philanthropic feeding resources often have inconsistent availability with limited hours and geographic distribution compared to government nutrition assistance programs and may be unable to provide the quantity and quality of food necessary for children or people with nutrition-sensitive health conditions. The relative scarcity of resources that are available and the difficulties that exist in actually accessing them underline the importance of providing ongoing support to families, in being persistent, and in having a well-designed and robust referral system in place that is kept up to date as changes occur in resource availability and eligibility.

The Importance of Advocacy

Physicians and other child health providers are in a vital position to advocate for their patients with FTT, both on individual and policy levels. Physicians or other team members who help connect individual patients with resources are advocating on their behalf, particularly in situations where resources are especially limited. Physicians may also be able to advocate for their low-income patients by interfacing with local community action agencies, which can help address unmet needs that could contribute to FTT [87].

Once they have been identified, the rectifying of unmet social needs relevant to FTT may fall outside the area of expertise of clinicians. For this reason, social determinants of FTT may sometimes be best addressed by the partnership of clinicians and lawyers. Specialist lawyers may be better equipped to advocate for patients directly to services they may qualify for, and to fight for the enforcement of health-promoting laws and regulations, such as housing codes [119]. In 1993, Boston Medical Center was among one of the first hospitals to integrate lawyers into its pediatric practice [120]. This program, now called the Medical–Legal Partnership, advises clinicians on how to assist the families of pediatric patients in domains including housing, immigration, family law, and health insurance [119]. The success of this program highlights the importance of involving experts in a variety of fields in the management of FTT through advocacy [119].

Advocacy on behalf of children at the policy level is also crucial. Policy-level advocacy targets specifically relevant to FTT include the design and distribution of government nutrition programs. A push to expand enrollment in SNAP, both through a widening of eligibility criteria and in making it easier to actually access the benefits, as well as increasing benefits to level approaching a more adequate diet can serve as an example of a way in which physicians can advocate on behalf of all low-income children—not just those with FTT. It is important for physicians and other health care professionals to use their expertise to educate policymakers on the connections between SDH and child health and development and health care and education costs [16].

The Grow Clinic: One Model for Multidisciplinary Treatment of Failure to Thrive

The Grow Clinic is an outpatient pediatric subspecialty clinic of Boston Medical Center, which was founded in 1984 to provide medical, nutritional, developmental, and social service assistance to children who are referred to the clinic with FTT. The Grow Clinic can thus be seen as one model of multidisciplinary care for children with FTT. The team treating each child consists of a pediatrician, dietitian, social worker, and a multilingual outreach worker [121]. Continuity of providers in each of these roles facilitates trust and the therapeutic alliance essential to facilitating recovery from FTT. Home visits are an integral part of care at the Grow Clinic, as they provide a clearer window into the social circumstances of each patient's family.

The Grow Clinic serves children under 5 years of age, and its patient population is profoundly impacted by negative social determinants of health [122]. To help mitigate the identified effects of food insecurity, a preventive food pantry was founded at Boston Medical Center. Initially intended to primarily serve the patients of the Grow Clinic, the program has expanded significantly since its founding in 2001 and now serves over 7000 people from all clinical services each month [123]. The Grow Clinic's model has reduced the admission rate for children it treats from 50% in 1984 to 5% in 2006 [122].

The inextricable link between FTT and social factors necessitates policy-focused research for evidence-based advocacy to advance the prevention and treatment of this condition. Children's HealthWatch (www.childrenshealthwatch.org) is a nonpartisan multicity network of Grow Clinic health providers, public health researchers, and policy experts dedicated to research and advocacy surrounding social and economic factors of children's health. Its research methods include repeat cross-sectional surveys of families with children aged below 4 years who present to one of five urban emergency departments and primary care clinics, focusing on identifying the potential health, growth, and developmental effects of SDH such as food insecurity, housing insecurity, and energy insecurity [124].

Afterword

Social determinants of health and their potential policy remedies are dynamic, changing with population-level health risks, socioeconomic conditions, and political will. Clinicians must ally with community agencies to keep current on these changes which have an immediate and persistent impact for good or ill on the families of children with growth faltering. After the text of this chapter was finalized, the COVID pandemic and consequent shutdowns dating from March 2020, increased the prevalence and severity of many of the SDH enumerated in this chapter. The burden of these pandemic conditions fell, as before, disproportionately on low-income families with children, particularly families of color and those with immigrant household members. As the coronavirus pandemic stretched on, millions of US children and their families faced food insecurity. With the closure of child care centers and schools during the first months of the pandemic, mothers with children were particularly burdened by the loss of employment and full-time child care responsibilities. Many families who were food secure before the onset of the pandemic became food insecure [125]. The Household Pulse survey found that households with children suffered higher levels of food and housing insecurity (behind on rent), compared to adult-only households. At Boston Medical Center the rate of referral of malnourished young children increased by 40% during the first year of the pandemic [126–128]. Pandemic EBT cards were introduced to replace food that children previously received at school or in child care. Universal free school meals were provided until the end of the 2021–2022 school year. The Child Tax Credit introduced in summer of 2021 briefly supported families' expenditures on food and housing resources, including many families who had previously been ineligible for the Earned Income Tax Credit because their incomes were so low that they were not required to file taxes. Unfortunately, payment of the child tax credit ended in December 2021. A moratorium on foreclosures and evictions which also ended in 2021 temporarily reduced the risk of family homelessness Unfortunately, most of these measures were temporary and have now expired or will do so at the end of the 2021–2022 school year.

Thus, clinicians must be alert to the impact on child growth and health of the recent withdrawal of resources from families presenting with a child whose growth is faltering. One responsibility of clinicians faced with these occurrences is to, within the bounds of professional confidentiality, document in the narrative details of the real-life consequences of policy changes on individual lives. Even deidentified case vignettes can contribute to powerful professional advocacy on behalf of children and families who otherwise have minimal input on policies and programs which influence their lives.

Clinical Cases

Case 1

History of Present Illness
A 2-year-old girl is brought to the clinic for a well-child check and is found to have a weight-for-age and weight-for-length below the third percentile, with a low rate of weight gain

when she was last seen in the office a year ago. She does not have any other known medical conditions.

Social History

A thorough social history reveals that the patient lives with her mother, they do not have stable housing, and have recently been in and out of local shelters. Over the past year, there have also been numerous occasions on which they ran out of food and did not have enough money to buy more.

What Is the Most Appropriate Course of Action?

In addition to nutritional counseling, the patient and her mother were referred to the clinic's in-house social worker, who worked with the city's housing authority to ensure stable placement in a shelter. The child and her mother will continue to follow up with the clinic social worker as the patient's mother applies for federal rental assistance and federal nutrition assistance programs. The patient's mother was also provided with a list of local food pantries for times of crisis.

Case 2

History of Present Illness

A 12-month-old boy with known FTT continues to show inadequate weight gain despite nutritional counseling with his parents, enrollment in SNAP, and negative laboratory testing. His parents demonstrate an understanding of their child's condition, as well as the ways in which it might be improved.

Social History

A more thorough social history reveals that the child's parents must both work beyond full time to support the family, and the patient and his two older siblings are supervised by their elderly maternal grandmother during this time.

What Might Be an Appropriate Course of Action?
With the permission of the child's parents, the clinic's social worker visits their home while the parents are at work and the children are in the care of their grandmother. The social worker speaks with the grandmother, who says that she feels overwhelmed at having to take care of the three children in part because of her own health issues. She finds herself giving the 12-month-old boy soda and fruit juice often when he is crying and she feels that she does not have time to prepare other food for him.

After her visit, the clinic's social worker makes a referral for the family to a state child care financial assistance agency with the hopes of providing access to childcare for at least the two older children so that the grandmother can give more attention to the 12-month-old boy. She also educates the grandmother on healthier feeding practices.

Key Points

- FTT in children is often associated with a complex series of interconnected social factors, many of which are downstream effects of poverty and financial stress
- Individual social determinants of health most relevant to FTT in children include food insecurity, housing instability, energy insecurity, and caregiver distress
- Participation in nutrition assistance programs has a beneficial effect on weight status in children and on parental depression
- The workup of children with suspected FTT should include the use of systematic screens for remediable negative social determinants of health
- An important treatment modality in the multidisciplinary care of FTT is referral to programs that facilitate access to adequate nutrition, housing, energy, childcare, and other essential needs; clinicians should become aware of what resources are available in their areas

More Information About Some of the Services and Programs Mentioned in This Chapter Can Be Obtained Through the Following Websites and Contact Numbers

Websites

- Supplemental Nutrition Assistance Program (SNAP) Online: A Review of State Government SNAP Websites

    - https://www.cbpp.org/research/snap-online-a-review-of-state-government-snap-websites?fa=view&id=618

- Contact information for state and local nutrition assistance programs/public health departments—includes Special Supplemental Nutrition Program for Women, Infants, and Children (WIC), Supplemental Nutrition Assistance Program (SNAP), and others

    - https://www.fns.usda.gov/contacts?f[0]=program%3A32

- Feeding America—includes directory of food banks searchable by ZIP Code

    - https://www.feedingamerica.org/

- Low Income Home Energy Assistance Program (LIHEAP)

    - https://www.acf.hhs.gov/ocs/programs/liheap

- Information on federal rental assistance programs.

    - https://www.cbpp.org/research/housing/policy-basics-federal-rental-assistance

- State and local lead screening programs

    - https://www.cdc.gov/nceh/lead/programs/default.htm

- Substance Abuse and Mental Health Services Administration (SAMHSA) Behavioral Health Treatment Services Locator

    - https://findtreatment.samhsa.gov/

- Children's HealthWatch
  - https://childrenshealthwatch.org/
- Screening tools
  - Well Child Care, Evaluation, Community Resources, Advocacy, Referral, Education (WE CARE): https://www.bmc.org/pediatrics-primary-care/we-care/we-care-model
  - Protocol for Responding to and Assessing Patients' Assets, Risks, and Experiences (PRAPARE): http://www.nachc.org/wp-content/uploads/2018/05/PRAPARE_One_Pager_Sept_2016.pdf
  - Health Related Social Needs (HRSN) Screening Tool: https://innovation.cms.gov/Files/worksheets/ahcm-screeningtool.pdf

Phone Numbers

- Supplemental Nutrition Assistance Program (SNAP) information line:
  - 1-800-221-5689
- Special Supplemental Nutrition Program for Women, Infants, and Children (WIC):
  - Varies by state: https://www.fns.usda.gov/wic/toll-free-numbers-wic-state-agencies
- National School Lunch Program (NSLP) customer service
  - 1-800-735-8778, ext. 6300
- Low Income Home Energy Assistance Program (LIHEAP):
  - 1-866-674-6327
- Housing and Urban Development (HUD) rental assistance counseling number
  - 1-800-569-4287

References

1. Krugman S, Dubowitz H. Failure to thrive. Am Fam Physician. 2003;68(5):879–84.
2. Coleman RW, Provence S. Environmental retardation (hospitalism) in infants living in families. Pediatrics. 1957;19(2):285–92.
3. Patton RG, Gardner LI. Influence of family environment on growth: the syndrome of "maternal deprivation." Pediatrics. 1962;30(6):957–62.
4. Garg A, Toy S, Tripodis Y, Silverstein M, Freeman E. Addressing social determinants of health at well child care visits: a cluster RCT. Pediatrics. 2015;135(2):e296–304.
5. Shi L, Macinko J, Starfield B, Xu J, Regan J, Politzer R, et al. Primary care, infant mortality, and low birth weight in the states of the USA. J Epidemiol Community Health. 2004;58(5):374–80.
6. Kelleher KJ, Casey PH, Bradley RH, Pope SK, Whiteside L, Barrett KW, et al. Risk factors and outcomes for failure to thrive in low birth weight preterm infants. Pediatrics. 1993;91(5):941–8.
7. Sices L, Wilson-Costello D, Minich N, Friedman H, Hack M. Postdischarge growth failure among extremely low birth weight infants: correlates and consequences. Paediatr Child Health. 2007;12(1):22–8.
8. Risnes KR, Vatten LJ, Baker JL, Jameson K, Sovio U, Kajantie E, et al. Birthweight and mortality in adulthood: a systematic review and meta-analysis. Int J Epidemiol. 2011;40(3):647–61.
9. Lau C, Ambalavanan N, Chakraborty H, Wingate MS, Carlo WA. Extremely low birth weight and infant mortality rates in the United States. Pediatrics. 2013;131(5):855–60.
10. World Health Organization. 2018 global reference list of 100 core health indicators (plus health-related SDGs) [Internet]. Geneva; 2018 [cited 2019 Nov 2]. Available from https://apps.who.int/iris/bitstream/handle/10665/259951/WHO-HIS-IER-GPM-2018.1-eng.pdf?sequence=1
11. Stoto M. Population health measurement: applying performance measurement concepts in population health settings. eGEMs. 2015;2(4):1132.
12. Stoto MA. Public health assessment in the 1990s. Annu Rev Public Health. 1992;13(1):59–78.
13. Casey PH. Growth of low birth weight preterm children. Semin Perinatol. 2008;32(1):20–7.

14. Hack M, Schluchter M, Cartar L, Rahman M, Cuttler L, Borawski E. Growth of very low birth weight infants to age 20 years. Pediatrics. 2003;112(1):e30–8.
15. Ross E, Munoz FM, Edem B, Nan C, Jehan F, Quinn J, et al. Failure to thrive: case definition & guidelines for data collection, analysis, and presentation of maternal immunisation safety data. Vaccine. 2017;35(48, Part A):6483–91.
16. Satcher D, Kaczorowski J, Topa D. The expanding role of the pediatrician in improving child health in the 21st century. Pediatrics. 2005;115(4):1124–8.
17. American Academy of Pediatrics: Committee on Nutrition. Failure to thrive. In: Kleinman R, editor. Pediatric nutrition handbook. 6th ed. Elk Grove Village, IL: American Academy of Pediatrics; 2008. p. 601–36.
18. Chaudry A, Wimer C. Poverty is not just an indicator: the relationship between income, poverty, and child well-being. Acad Pediatr. 2016;16(3):S23–9.
19. Schenck-Fontaine A, Panico L. Many kinds of poverty: three dimensions of economic hardship, their combinations, and children's behavior problems. Demography. 2019;56(6):2279–305.
20. Pascoe JM, Wood DL, Duffee JH, Kuo A. Mediators and adverse effects of child poverty in the United States. Pediatrics. 2016;137(4):e20160340.
21. Cook JT, Frank DA. Food security, poverty, and human development in the United States. Ann N Y Acad Sci. 2008;1136(1):193–209.
22. Coleman-Jensen A, Rabbitt MP, Gregory CA, Singh A. Household Food Security in the United States in 2020. 2021 [cited 2022 Jan 15]; Available from www.ers.usda.gov
23. Winicki J, Jemison K. Food insecurity and hunger in the kindergarten classroom: its effect on learning and growth. Contemp Econ Policy. 2003;21(2):145–57.
24. Zhu Y, Mangini LD, Hayward MD, Forman MR. Food insecurity and the extremes of childhood weight: defining windows of vulnerability. Int J Epidemiol. 2019;49(2):1–9.
25. Cook JT, Frank DA, Berkowitz C, Black MM, Casey PH, Cutts DB, et al. Food insecurity is associated with adverse health outcomes among human infants and toddlers. J Nutr. 2004;134(6):1432–8.
26. Kirkpatrick SI, McIntyre L, Potestio ML. Child hunger and long-term adverse consequences for health. Arch Pediatr Adolesc Med. 2010;164(8):754–62.

27. Skalicky A, Meyers AF, Adams WG, Yang Z, Cook JT, Frank DA. Child food insecurity and iron deficiency anemia in low-income infants and toddlers in the United States. Matern Child Health J. 2006;10(2):177–85.

28. Ryu JH, Bartfeld JS. Household food insecurity during childhood and subsequent health status: the Early Childhood Longitudinal Study—Kindergarten Cohort. Am J Public Health. 2012;102(11):e50–5.

29. Howard LL. Does food insecurity at home affect non-cognitive performance at school? A longitudinal analysis of elementary student classroom behavior. Econ Educ Rev. 2011;30(1):157–76.

30. Casey P, Goolsby S, Berkowitz C, Frank D, Cook J, Cutts D, et al. Maternal depression, changing public assistance, food security, and child health status. Pediatrics. 2004;113(2):298–304.

31. Cutts DB, Coleman S, Black MM, Chilton MM, Cook JT, de Cuba SE, et al. Homelessness during pregnancy: a unique, time-dependent risk factor of birth outcomes. Matern Child Health J. 2015;19(6):1276–83.

32. Carrion BV, Earnshaw VA, Kershaw T, Lewis JB, Stasko EC, Tobin JN, et al. Housing instability and birth weight among young urban mothers. J Urban Health. 2015;92(1):1–9.

33. Sandel M, Sheward R, De Cuba SE, Coleman SM, Frank DA, Chilton M, et al. Unstable housing and caregiver and child health in renter families. Pediatrics. 2018;141(2):e20172199.

34. Lanphear BP, Roghmann KJ. Pathways of lead exposure in urban children. Environ Res. 1997;74(1):67–73.

35. Jones R, Homa D, Meyer P, Brody D, Caldwell K, Pirkle J, et al. Trends in blood lead levels and blood lead testing among US children aged 1 to 5 years, 1988–2004. Pediatrics. 2009;123(3):e376–85.

36. Jacobs DE, Clickner RP, Zhou JY, Viet SM, Marker DA, Rogers JW, et al. The prevalence of lead-based paint hazards in U.S. housing. Environ Health Perspect. 2002;110(10):A599–606.

37. Hanna-Attisha M, LaChance J, Sadler RC, Schnepp AC. Elevated blood lead levels in children associated with the Flint drinking water crisis: a spatial analysis of risk and public health response. Am J Public Health. 2016;106(2):283–90.

38. Kwong WT, Friello P, Semba RD. Interactions between iron deficiency and lead poisoning: epidemiology and pathogenesis. Sci Total Environ. 2004;330(1–3):21–37.

39. Bithoney WG. Elevated lead levels in children with nonorganic failure to thrive. Pediatrics. 1986;78(5):891–5.

40. Council on Environmental Health. Prevention of childhood lead toxicity. Pediatrics. 2016;138(1):e20161493.
41. Hernández D. Understanding 'energy insecurity' and why it matters to health. Soc Sci Med. 2016;167:1–10.
42. Frank DA, Roos N, Meyers A, Napoleone M, Peterson K, Cather A, et al. Seasonal variation in weight-for-age in a pediatric emergency room. Public Health Rep. 1996;111(4):366–71.
43. Bhattacharya J, DeLeire T, Haider S, Currie J. Heat or eat? Cold-weather shocks and nutrition in poor American families. Am J Public Health. 2003;93(7):1149–54.
44. Jhun I, Mata D, Nordio F, Lee M, Schwartz J, Zanobetti A. Ambient temperature and sudden infant death syndrome in the United States. Epidemiology. 2017;28(5):728–34.
45. Zhang Y, Yu C, Wang L. Temperature exposure during pregnancy and birth outcomes: an updated systematic review of epidemiological evidence. Environ Pollut. 2017;225:700–12.
46. Cook J, Frank D, Casey P, Rose-Jacobs R. A brief indicator of household energy security: associations with food security, child health, and child development in US infants and toddlers. Pediatrics. 2008;122(4):e867–75.
47. Jaffe AC. Failure to thrive: current clinical concepts. Pediatr Rev. 2011;32(3):100–8.
48. Lorant V, Deliège D, Eaton W, Robert A, Philippot P, Ansseau M. Socioeconomic inequalities in depression: a meta-analysis. Am J Epidemiol. 2003;157(2):98–112.
49. Assari S. Social determinants of depression: the intersections of race, gender, and socioeconomic status. Brain Sci. 2017;7(12):156.
50. O'Brien LM, Heycock EG, Hanna M, Jones PW, Cox JL. Postnatal depression and faltering growth: a community study. Pediatrics. 2004;113(5):1242–7.
51. Wojcicki JM, Holbrook K, Lustig RH, Epel E, Caughey AB, Muñoz RF, et al. Chronic maternal depression is associated with reduced weight gain in Latino infants from birth to 2 years of age. PLoS One. 2011;6(2):e16737.
52. Surkan PJ, Kennedy CE, Hurley KM, Black MM. Maternal depression and early childhood growth in developing countries: systematic review and meta-analysis. Bull World Health Organ. 2011;89(8):608–15.
53. Grote V, Vik T, von Kries R, Luque V, Socha J, Verduci E, et al. Maternal postnatal depression and child growth: a European cohort study. BMC Pediatr. 2010;10(1):14.

54. Stewart RC. Maternal depression and infant growth—a review of recent evidence. Matern Child Nutr. 2007;3(2):94–107.

55. Drewett RF, Blair P, Emmett P, Emond A. Failure to thrive in the term and preterm infants of mothers depressed in the postnatal period: a population-based birth cohort study. J Child Psychol Psychiatry Allied Discip. 2004;45(2):359–66.

56. Wright C, Birks E. Risk factors for failure to thrive: a population-based survey. Child Care Health Dev. 2000;26(1):5–16.

57. Block R, Krebs N. Failure to thrive as a manifestation of child neglect. Pediatrics. 2005;116(5):1234–7.

58. Black MM, Dubowitz H, Casey PH, Cutts D, Drewett R, Drotar D, et al. Failure to thrive as distinct from child neglect. Pediatrics. 2006;117(4):1456–8.

59. De Jong RB, Bekhof J, Roorda R, Zwart P. Severe nutritional vitamin deficiency in a breast-fed infant of a vegan mother. Eur J Pediatr. 2005;164(4):259–60.

60. Kühne T, Bubl R, Baumgartner R. Maternal vegan diet causing a serious infantile neurological disorder due to vitamin B 12 deficiency. Eur J Pediatr. 1991;150(3):205–8.

61. Smith MM, Lifshitz F. Excess fruit juice consumption as a contributing factor in nonorganic failure to thrive. Pediatrics. 1994;93(3):438–43.

62. Heyman MB, Abrams SA. Fruit juice in infants, children, and adolescents: current recommendations. Pediatrics. 2017;139(6):e20170967.

63. Spencer NJ. Failure to think about failure to thrive. Arch Dis Child. 2007;92(2):95–6.

64. Blair PS, Drewett RF, Emmett PM, Ness A, Emond AM. Family, socioeconomic and prenatal factors associated with failure to thrive in the Avon longitudinal study of parents and children (ALSPAC). Int J Epidemiol. 2004;33(4):839–47.

65. Abdelhadi RA, Bouma S, Bairdain S, Wolff J, Legro A, Plogsted S, et al. Characteristics of hospitalized children with a diagnosis of malnutrition: United States, 2010. J Parenter Enter Nutr. 2016;40(5):623–35.

66. Miller JE, Korenman S. Poverty and children's nutritional status in the United States. Am J Epidemiol. 1994;140(3):233–43.

67. Frederick CB, Snellman K, Putnam RD. Increasing socioeconomic disparities in adolescent obesity. PNAS. 2014;111(4):1338–42.

68. Drewnowski A, Specter SE. Poverty and obesity: the role of energy density and energy costs. Am J Clin Nutr. 2004;79(1):6–16.

69. Lee BJ, Mackey-Bilaver L. Effects of WIC and Food Stamp Program participation on child outcomes. Child Youth Serv Rev. 2007;29(4):501–17.
70. Owen AL, Owen GM. Twenty years of WIC: a review of some effects of the program. J Am Diet Assoc. 1997;97(7):777–82.
71. Black MM, Cutts DB, Frank DA, Geppert J, Skalicky A, Levenson S, et al. Special Supplemental Nutrition Program for Women, Infants, and Children participation and infants' growth and health: a multisite surveillance study. Pediatrics. 2004;114(1):169–76.
72. Bitler MP, Currie J. Does WIC work? The effects of WIC on pregnancy and birth outcomes. J Policy Anal Manag. 2005;24(1):73–91.
73. Kowaleski-Jones L, Duncan GJ. Effects of participation in the WIC program on birthweight: evidence from the National Longitudinal Survey of Youth. Am J Public Health. 2002;92(5):799–804.
74. Sonchak L. The impact of WIC on birth outcomes: new evidence from South Carolina. Matern Child Health J. 2016;20(7):1518–25.
75. Metcoff J, Costiloe P, Crosby WM, Dutta S, Sandstead HH, Milne D, et al. Effect of food supplementation (WIC) during pregnancy on birth weight. Am J Clin Nutr. 1985;41(5):933–47.
76. Fingar KR, Lob SH, Dove MS, Gradziel P, Curtis MP. Reassessing the association between WIC and birth outcomes using a fetuses-at-risk approach. Matern Child Health J. 2017;21(4):825–35.
77. Arteaga I, Heflin C, Gable S. The impact of aging out of WIC on food security in households with children. Child Youth Serv Rev. 2016;69:82–96.
78. Almond D, Hoynes HW, Schanzenbach DW. Inside the war on poverty: the impact of food stamps on birth outcomes. Rev Econ Stat. 2011;93(2):387–403.
79. Ettinger de Cuba SA, Bovell-Ammon AR, Cook JT, Coleman SM, Black MM, Chilton MM, et al. SNAP, young children's health, and family food security and healthcare access. Am J Prev Med. 2019;57(4):525–32.
80. Ratcliffe C, McKernan SM, Zhang S. How much does the supplemental nutrition assistance program reduce food insecurity? Am J Agric Econ. 2011;93(4):1082–98.
81. Mabli J, Ohls J. Supplemental Nutrition Assistance Program participation is associated with an increase in household food security in a national evaluation. J Nutr. 2015;145(2):344–51.

82. Korenman S, Abner KS, Kaestner R, Gordon RA. The child and adult care food program and the nutrition of preschoolers. Early Child Res Q. 2013;28(2):325–36.
83. U.S. Department of Agriculture Food and Nutrition Service. Program Information Report (Keydata)—US Summary, FY 2021 [Internet]. 2021 Oct [cited 2022 Jan 15]. Available from https://fns-prod.azureedge.net/sites/default/files/data-files/keydata-october-2021.pdf
84. Perl L. LIHEAP: program and funding [Internet]. 2018 [cited 2019 Nov 19]. Available from https://fas.org/sgp/crs/misc/RL31865.pdf
85. US Department of Health and Human Services Administration for Children and Families. LOW INCOME HOME ENERGY ASSISTANCE PROGRAM Report to Congress for Fiscal Year 2015 [Internet]. 2016 [cited 2022 Jan 16]. Available from http://www.acf.hhs.gov/programs/ocs/programs/liheap
86. Wein O. The Low Income Home Energy Assistance Program (LIHEAP) [Internet]. 2017 [cited 2019 Dec 7]. Available from https://www.https//nlihc.org/sites/default/files/AG-2017/2017AG_Ch05-S08_Low-Income-Home-Energy-Assistance-Program_LIHEAP.pdf
87. Frank DA, Neault NB, Skalicky A, Cook JT, Wilson JD, Levenson S, et al. Heat or eat: the Low Income Home Energy Assistance Program and nutritional and health risks among children less than 3 years of age. Pediatrics. 2006;118(5):e1293–302.
88. Meyers A, Cutts D, Frank DA, Levenson S, Skalicky A, Heeren T, et al. Subsidized housing and children's nutritional status: data from a multisite surveillance study. Arch Pediatr Adolesc Med. 2005;159(6):551–6.
89. WIC eligibility requirements. USDA-FNS [Internet]. [cited 2019 Nov 20]. Available from https://www.fns.usda.gov/wic/wic-eligibility-requirements
90. Child nutrition programs: income eligibility guidelines [Internet]. 2019 [cited 2020 Jan 12]. Available from https://www.fns.usda.gov/cnp/fr-032019
91. Smith A, Tiehen L. Participation in SNAP varies across states but is generally decreasing [Internet]. 2019 [cited 2019 Nov 5]. Available from https://www.ers.usda.gov/amber-waves/2018/september/participation-in-snap-varies-across-states-but-is-generally-decreasing/
92. Center on Budget and Policy Priorities. A quick guide to SNAP eligibility and benefits [Internet]. [cited 2019

Nov 5]. Available from https://www.cbpp.org/research/food-assistance/a-quick-guide-to-snap-eligibility-and-benefits

93. Aussenberg RA, Falk G. The Supplemental Nutrition Assistance Program (SNAP): categorical eligibility [Internet]. 2017 [cited 2019 Nov 5]. Available from http://www.nationalaglawcenter.org/wp-content/uploads/assets/crs/R42054.pdf

94. Cunnyngham K. Reaching Those in Need: estimates of State Supplemental Nutrition Assistance Program Participation Rates in 2018 [Internet]. Alexandria, VA; 2021 [cited 2022 Jan 16]. Available from https://fns-prod.azureedge.net/sites/default/files/resource-files/Reaching2018-Summary.pdf

95. Newman C, Scherpf E. Supplemental Nutrition Assistance Program (SNAP) access at the state and county Levels: evidence from Texas SNAP administrative records and the American Community Survey, ERR-156 [Internet]. 2013 [cited 2019 Nov 5]. Available from https://www.ers.usda.gov/webdocs/publications/45136/40264_err-156_summary.pdf?v=42642

96. Pinard CA, Bertmann FMW, Byker Shanks C, Schober DJ, Smith TM, Carpenter LC, et al. What factors influence SNAP participation? Literature reflecting enrollment in food assistance programs from a social and behavioral science perspective. J Hunger Environ Nutr. 2017;12(2):151–68.

97. National Immigration Forum. Fact sheet: immigrants and public benefits [Internet]. [cited 2019 Sep 11]. Available from https://immigrationforum.org/article/fact-sheet-immigrants-and-public-benefits/

98. Broder T, Moussavian A, Blazer J. Overview of immigrant eligibility for federal programs [Internet]. 2015 [cited 2019 Sep 11]. Available from https://www.nilc.org/issues/economic-support/overview-immeligfedprograms/

99. United States Department of Agriculture—Food and Nutrition Service. SNAP Policy on non-citizen eligibility [Internet]. 2013 [cited 2019 Sep 11]. Available from https://www.fns.usda.gov/snap/eligibility/citizen/non-citizen-policy

100. Bovell-Ammon A, Ettinger De Cuba S, Coleman S, Ahmad N, Black MM, Frank DA, et al. Trends in food insecurity and SNAP participation among immigrant families of U.S.-born young children. Children. 2019;6(4):55.

101. Dewey C. Immigrants are going hungry so Trump won't deport them. The Washington Post [Internet]. 2017 Mar 16 [cited 2019 Oct 28]; Available from https://www.washingtonpost.com/news/

wonk/wp/2017/03/16/immigrants-are-now-canceling-their-food-stamps-for-fear-that-trump-will-deport-them/

102. Quandt SA, Shoaf JI, Tapia J, Hernández-Pelletier M, Clark HM, Arcury TA. Experiences of Latino immigrant families in North Carolina help explain elevated levels of food insecurity and hunger. J Nutr. 2006;136(10):2638–44.

103. Potochnick S, Chen JH, Perreira K. Local-level immigration enforcement and food insecurity risk among Hispanic immigrant families with children: national-level evidence. J Immigr Minor Health. 2017;19(5):1042–9.

104. Chung EK, Siegel BS, Garg A, Conroy K, Gross RS, Long DA, et al. Screening for social determinants of health among children and families living in poverty: a guide for clinicians. Curr Probl Pediatr Adolesc Health Care. 2016;46(5):135–53.

105. The WE CARE Model. Boston Medical Center [Internet]. [cited 2019 Dec 2]. Available from https://www.bmc.org/pediatrics-primary-care/we-care/we-care-model

106. Hager ER, Quigg AM, Black MM, Coleman SM, Heeren T, Rose-Jacobs R, et al. Development and validity of a 2-item screen to identify families at risk for food insecurity. Pediatrics. 2010;126(1):e26–32.

107. Gottlieb L, Hessler D, Long D, Amaya A, Adler N. A randomized trial on screening for social determinants of health: the iScreen study. Pediatrics. 2014;134(6):e1611–8.

108. Alley DE, Asomugha CN, Conway PH, Sanghavi DM. Accountable Health Communities—addressing social needs through medicare and medicaid. N Engl J Med. 2016;374(1):8–11.

109. Accountable Health Communities Model. Center for Medicare & Medicaid Innovation [Internet]. [cited 2019 Dec 2]. Available from https://innovation.cms.gov/initiatives/ahcm

110. PRAPARE: Protocol for Responding to and Assessing Patient Assets, Risks, and Experiences [Internet]. 2016 [cited 2019 Dec 2]. Available from www.nachc.org/PRAPARE

111. United States Department of Agriculture—Economic Research Service. Survey Tools [Internet] 2019 [cited 2019 Oct 24]. Available from https://www.ers.usda.gov/topics/food-nutrition-assistance/food-security-in-the-us/survey-tools/

112. American Academy of Pediatrics Council on Community Pediatrics Committee on Nutrition. Promoting food security for all children. Pediatrics. 2015;136(5):e1431–8.

113. Gattu R, Paik G, Wang Y, Ray P, Lichenstein R, Black MM. The Hunger Vital Sign identifies household food insecurity among children in emergency departments and primary care. Children. 2019;6(10):107.
114. Stout S, Klucznik C, Chevalier A, Wheeler R, Azzara J, Gray L, et al. Cambridge Health Alliance model of team-based care implementation guide and toolkit. [cited 2019 Oct 23]; Available from www.ihi.org
115. Next Steps in Care. Referring patients and family caregivers to community-based services: a provider's guide [Internet]. 2013 [cited 2019 Oct 23]. Available from https://www.nextstepin-care.org/uploads/File/Guides/Provider/Community_Based_Services.pdf
116. Aunt Bertha—connecting people and programs [Internet]. [cited 2019 Nov 9]. Available from https://www.auntbertha.com/
117. Home—CharityTracker from Simon Solutions [Internet]. [cited 2019 Nov 9]. Available from https://www.charitytracker.net/
118. Cartier Y, Fichtenberg C, Gottlieb L. Community resource referral platforms: a guide for health care organizations [Internet]. 2019 [cited 2019 Oct 23]. Available from https://sirenetwork.ucsf.edu/sites/sirenetwork.ucsf.edu/files/wysiwyg/Community-Resource-Referral-Platforms-Guide.pdf
119. Zuckerman B, Sandel M, Smith L, Lawton E. Why pediatricians need lawyers to keep children healthy. Pediatrics. 2004;114(1):224–8.
120. Goldberg C. Boston Medical Center turns to lawyers for a cure. The New York Times [Internet]. 2001 May 16 [cited 2019 Oct 23]; Available from https://www.nytimes.com/2001/05/16/us/boston-medical-center-turns-to-lawyers-for-a-cure.html
121. Grow Clinic at BMC [Internet]. [cited 2019 Nov 9]. Available from http://www.bu.edu/womensguild/files/2018/11/207_Ped_Grow-Clinic-Brochure-to-email.pdf
122. Grow Clinic. Boston Medical Center [Internet]. [cited 2019 Nov 9]. Available from https://dev.bmc.org/programs/grow-clinic
123. AHA News. Boston Medical Center makes healthy food part of patients' medical care [Internet]. 2017 [cited 2019 Nov 10]. Available from https://www.aha.org/news/headline/2017-10-12-boston-medical-center-makes-healthy-food-part-patients--medical-care
124. Children's HealthWatch—Home [Internet]. [cited 2019 Nov 10]. Available from https://childrenshealthwatch.org/

125. Morales DX, Morales SA, Beltran TF. Food Insecurity in Households with Children Amid the COVID-19 Pandemic: evidence from the Household Pulse Survey: https://doi.org/101177/23294965211011593 [Internet]. 2021 Apr 23 [cited 2022 Jan 16];8(4):314–25. Available from https://journals.sage-pub.com/doi/full/10.1177/23294965211011593

126. Fleischhacker S, Bleich S. Addressing food insecurity in the United States during and after the COVID-19 pandemic: the role of the Federal Nutrition Safety Net. J Food Law Policy [Internet] 2021 Sep 27 [cited 2022 Jan 16];17(1). Available from https://scholarworks.uark.edu/jflp/vol17/iss1/8

127. Priorities C on B and P. Tracking the COVID-19 Economy's Effects on Food, Housing, and Employment Hardships [Internet]. [cited 2022 Jan 16]. Available from https://www.cbpp.org/research/poverty-and-inequality/tracking-the-covid-19-economys-effects-on-food-housing-and

128. Kerr E. When COVID relief measures expire and how to prepare. Family Finance. US News [Internet]. US News & World Report. 2021 [cited 2022 Jan 16]. Available from https://money.usnews.com/money/personal-finance/family-finance/articles/when-covid-relief-measures-expire-and-how-to-prepare

Chapter 7
Improvement Opportunities for Practitioners: Developing a Clinical Pathway

Gerd McGwire, Ann-Marie Tantoco, and Allison Heacock

Introduction

Failure to thrive (FTT) can present as weight loss, failure to gain weight, or suboptimal growth, with the etiology often being multifactorial and related to the age of the child. With some exceptions, the care of a child with FTT can usually be managed in the outpatient setting but it remains a common reason for hospital admission for children less than 24 months of age [1]. There is no national guideline and few quality studies to guide providers regarding best practice for these

G. McGwire (✉) · A. Heacock
Section of Hospital Pediatrics, Nationwide Children's Hospital and The Ohio State University, Columbus, OH, USA
e-mail: Gerd.McGwire@nationwidechildrens.org;
Allison.Heacock@nationwidechildrens.org

A.-M. Tantoco
Department of Hospital Based Medicine, Ann & Robert H. Lurie Children's Hospital of Chicago and Northwestern University, Chicago, IL, USA
e-mail: attantoco@luriechildrens.org

© Springer Nature Switzerland AG 2023
J. G. Vachani (ed.), *Failure to Thrive and Malnutrition*,
https://doi.org/10.1007/978-3-031-14164-5_7

patients. An institutional FTT guideline or pathway can be helpful to align care between the outpatient and inpatient setting, decrease the use of ineffective tests and treatments, decrease unnecessary variation in care, increase efficiency of care, and improve outcome of patients admitted for FTT.

Case Study[1]

A hospital pediatrics service at a large freestanding pediatric hospital noted that FTT was the fifth most common diagnosis code. Upon further analysis, the length of stay (LOS) and readmission rates for these patients were noted to be higher than for patients with other conditions managed on the service. Discussions revealed that management practices varied widely among providers. A multidisciplinary team was assembled to develop a clinical pathway and QI initiatives to improve quality of care, decrease unwarranted variability, and optimize efficiency and resource utilization while decreasing risk of readmission for FTT patients.

Clinical Pathway Development

General Concepts

A clinical pathway is a structured multidisciplinary plan of care that translates guidelines, evidence, and expert opinion into localized infrastructure and processes [2]. Pathways detail the steps of clinical care in an algorithm or other "inventory of actions." The goal is to guide providers in the evaluation and treatment of a particular population or clinical condition [2]. A wide range of pediatric pathways as well as descriptions of pathway development methodology are now publicly available [3–5]. A pathway commonly provides

---

1Case Study is based off actual work performed by a team at Nationwide Children's Hospital, Columbus, Ohio

clinical tools to help close the gap between existing evidence and real-time clinical decision-making. The aim of pathways is to improve quality of care through the standardization of management based on evidence in published medical literature and/or expert opinion. Standardization should facilitate a reduction in variability in care among providers while allowing for customization based on individual patient needs and circumstances.

Clinical pathways facilitate continued quality improvement efforts by defining best practice and standardizing care. They are living documents that should be adapted continuously to improve care by incorporating new evidence as well as results from measurement [4].

Assembling the Team

A multidisciplinary team is central to the development of most pathways but particularly important for FTT. Team members representing all stakeholders in the care of these patients should contribute their expertise in the development of the pathway as well as facilitate its implementation in their area of practice once it is completed. In addition, each team should have an executive sponsor or committee that provides needed resources and oversight. Data analysts and project management representation are also helpful to assist clinical providers with design, data analysis, and organization.

Pearls

- Due to the multifactorial causation and paucity of high-quality evidence on FTT, a multi- and interdisciplinary team with expertise in all areas of pediatric feeding and growth, as well as a parent representative is pivotal to the successful development of an FTT pathway.

- Close cooperation between inpatient and outpatient providers is needed to align outpatient and inpatient management of FTT and to optimize awareness of and adherence to recommended admission criteria across the continuum of care.

Pathway Criteria and Definitions

The first step in pathway development is to define the condition or diagnosis. Diagnostic criteria for FTT are especially challenging as has been discussed in other chapters of this book. For pathway purposes, teams can use any or all of the available criteria including weight for age or length, weight for desirable (median) weight for age or lengths, deceleration of growth velocity, and weight gain per day or triceps skinfold thickness [6–10]. Documentation of malnutrition may be required for reimbursement of a hospitalization; including criteria for malnutrition severity in the pathway will likely improve documentation accuracy.

Next, teams should determine pathway inclusion and exclusion criteria, i.e., "To which patient does this pathway apply?" Factors to consider for FTT inclusion and exclusion criteria include age, past medical history, and medical stability. Although FTT is most commonly managed in the outpatient setting, failed outpatient management and concerning parent–child circumstances may warrant inpatient admission for diagnostic evaluation and the development of an effective care plan. Another factor to consider is whether the pathway will apply to repeat admissions for FTT or just the first episode of care.

Outlining Current Practice

To identify key management decisions as well as targets for improvement such as areas with ineffective care, large variations in care, or high resource utilization, it is important to outline current practice completely and accurately. This should include care provided by physicians, nurses, ancillary care providers, and any other stakeholders. Good communication between providers and staff is paramount to identify improvement opportunities. Construction of a flow chart will provide visualization. Specific targets for FTT care improvement can include when to obtain diagnostic lab tests and imaging, determining optimal frequency and techniques for feedings and weight measurements, and the involvement of consultants in care.

Evidence Review

A comprehensive literature review can be time consuming and should begin with a search to find existing pathways, national guidelines, or a synthesis of evidence such as systematic reviews and meta-analyses. A search for additional evidence should be guided by specific clinical questions that arise in the analysis of current practice. Questions should be defined in terms of Population, Intervention, Comparison, and Outcome (PICO) to identify keywords for the literature search. Examples of keywords for FTT include failure to thrive, malnutrition, weight faltering, FTT, and weight gain. Consulting a librarian for assistance is recommended. Members of the development team should review the collected evidence and make recommendations about care based on their findings and assessment. Assistance by experts in evidence-based medicine is helpful but may not be available. The GRADE methodology is the nationally adopted system used to rate evidence and develop recommendations for care [11]. For clinical questions with no or insufficient evidence, expert opinions may be solicited and care recommendations developed by team consensus.

Pearls

- Time constraints can be managed by a sequential search and review of evidence starting with existing pathways, national guidelines, systematic reviews, and meta-analyses followed by a review of lower quality evidence only if necessary.

Pitfalls

- When constructing a flow chart of current practice, care must be taken to ensure stakeholders create the document map only within their area of care rather than assuming knowledge of another team's systems or processes.

Management Algorithm

A management algorithm should include key steps in care, especially where a change in practice is anticipated. An algorithm for FTT management should start with outpatient care to indicate whether emergency department (ED) evaluation or direct admission is appropriate and continue through inpatient care and discharge. Recommended monitoring as well as criteria for severity assessment are usually included. A list of clinical findings suggestive of patient deterioration are helpful to optimize situational awareness and provide guidance to prevent unexpected clinical decompensation. Discharge planning and adequate follow-up should be outlined to optimize efficiency, decrease length of stay, and potentially prevent readmission.

Pearls

- Using a standardized format for an institution's pathway algorithms allows providers to quickly recognize key care items.

Best Practice Recommendations

Information to consider for an FTT pathway includes pertinent history or exam items, differential diagnosis, recommended assessments and monitoring, definitions of malnutrition, indications for ED referral or admission, involvement of ancillary services and specialty physicians, recommendations for diagnostic testing and treatments as well as tests and treatments that are not beneficial and, finally, discharge criteria with discharge planning, including caregiver education. Further details about best practice recommendations are included below to clarify and expand on the algorithm.

Clinical Support Tools

Electronic Medical Record (EMR) tools are usually needed to operationalize a pathway, with evidence-based order sets most commonly used to implement recommended care into clinical practice. In addition, best practice advisories and note templates can be helpful to increase awareness of recommended care and to facilitate documentation of the pathway decision-making process.

Pearls

- Use of an order set or similar EMR tool is often used to determine which patients are "on pathway."

Case Study Update

To reduce unwarranted variation in care, optimize resource utilization, decrease readmission rate, and improve overall patient outcomes, we developed a clinical pathway for inpatient management of FTT. A team was formed consisting of a primary care pediatrician, pediatric hospitalists, a pediatric emergency medicine physician, pediatric subspecialists from gastroenterology and neonatology, pediatric residents, representatives from care coordination/case management, social work (SW), nursing, occupational therapy (OT), a lactation consultant, a registered dietitian (RD), and a QI project coordinator. We formulated inclusion and exclusion criteria for the age range of patients most commonly admitted to our institution for FTT. Children with a previously diagnosed chronic medical condition or a previous hospital admission for FTT at our institution were excluded from the pathway.

- Inclusion criteria: Children <24 months of age were admitted to the hospital with suspected failure to thrive
- Exclusion criteria: Children ≥24 months of age, children with a known medical disorder that can cause growth delay, previous hospital admission for FTT
- FTT was diagnosed using one or more of the following criteria [6, 12–17]:

    - Weight for age < 5th percentile on a standard WHO growth chart 0–24 months
    - Weight-for-length < 5th percentile on a standard WHO growth chart 0–24 months
    - Weight is less than 90% of the desirable weight (desirable weight = corresponding 50th percentile weight for the patient's length on weight-for-length chart)
    - Deceleration of growth velocity across two major percentile lines and/or decrease of more than 2 standard deviations on a CDC or WHO growth chart over a period of 3–6 months

Current practice was outlined by the multidisciplinary team using a process map. The team then determined key clinical decision points and identified areas of large practice variation, high resource utilization, and inefficiency in care. PICO questions were used for evidence assessment including a search of the literature from 1990 to present and for a population of 0–5 years of age.

PICO questions with sufficient evidence available for management recommendations:

1. In children <24 months admitted with failure to thrive, does obtain screening lab work compared to obtaining labs based on suspected diagnoses lead to underlying diagnosis of failure to thrive?
2. In children <24 months admitted with failure to thrive, does further evaluation from SW compared to basic SW psychosocial screen lead to better outcomes?

3. In children <24 months admitted with failure to thrive, what are the appropriate admission criteria?
4. In patients admitted with failure to thrive, who are at risk for refeeding syndrome?
5. What frequency of labs should be obtained in a patient at risk for refeeding syndrome?
6. Does the use of a multidisciplinary team improve outcomes?

PICO questions with insufficient evidence; management recommendations solely based on team consensus:

1. In children <24 months admitted with failure to thrive, what are the appropriate discharge criteria?
2. Is there evidence that patients admitted with failure to thrive should gain weight prior to hospital discharge?
3. Is there a way to recognize oral-motor inefficiencies in FTT?
4. Is there evidence to support the use of 24-h caregiver care prior to discharge of FTT patients?
5. Does addition of a multivitamin in a patient with FTT improve growth?

The team developed a management algorithm incorporating evidence- and consensus-based care recommendations (Fig. 7.1).

Further details about best practice recommendations:

- History must include:

    - Feeding history
    - Developmental history
    - Past medical history—include pregnancy and birth history, birth weight
    - Family history—include systemic diseases, poor growth, and short stature
    - Psychosocial history—include primary caregivers and who live at home
    - Detailed review of systems—include gastrointestinal symptoms, stool production, respiratory issues, and recurrent infection

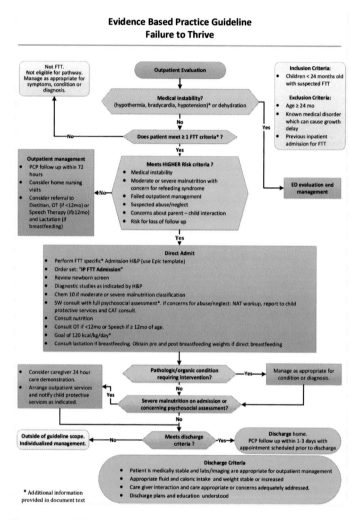

Evidence Based Practice Guideline
Failure to Thrive

Outpatient Evaluation

Not FTT.
Not eligible for pathway.
Manage as appropriate for
symptoms, condition or
diagnosis.

Medical instability?
(hypothermia, bradycardia, hypotension)* or dehydration

No

Does patient meet ≥ 1 FTT criteria* ?

Yes

Inclusion Criteria:
- Children < 24 months old
  with suspected FTT

Exclusion Criteria:
- Age ≥ 24 mo
- Known medical disorder
  which can cause growth
  delay
- Previous inpatient
  admission for FTT

Meets HIGHER Risk criteria ?
- Medical instability
- Moderate or severe malnutrition with
  concern for refeeding syndrome
- Failed outpatient management
- Suspected abuse/neglect
- Concerns about parent – child interaction
- Risk for loss of follow up

Outpatient management
- PCP follow up within 72
  hours
- Consider home nursing
  visits
- Consider referral to
  Dietitian, OT (if <12mo) or
  Speech Therapy (if≥12mo)
  and Lactation (if
  breastfeeding)

ED evaluation and
management

Yes

Direct Admit
- Perform FTT specific* Admission H&P (use Epic template)
- Order set: "IP FTT Admission"
- Review newborn screen
- Diagnostic studies as indicated by H&P
- Chem 10 if moderate or severe malnutrition classification
- SW consult with full psychosocial assessment*. If concerns for abuse/neglect: NAT workup, report to child
  protective services and CAT consult.
- Consult nutrition
- Consult OT if <12mo or Speech if ≥ 12mo of age.
- Goal of 120 kcal/kg/day*
- Consult lactation if breastfeeding. Obtain pre and post breastfeeding weights if direct breastfeeding

- Consider caregiver 24 hour
  care demonstration.
- Arrange outpatient services
  and notify child protective
  services as indicated.

Pathologic/organic condition
requiring intervention?

Yes

Manage as appropriate for
condition or diagnosis.

No

Yes

Severe malnutrition on admission or
concerning psychosocial assessment?

No

Outside of guideline scope.
Individualized management.

No

Meets discharge
criteria ?

Yes

Discharge home.
PCP follow up in 1-3 days with
appointment scheduled prior to discharge

Discharge Criteria
- Patient is medically stable and labs/imaging are appropriate for outpatient management
- Appropriate fluid and caloric intake and weight stable or increased
- Care giver interaction and care appropriate or concerns adequately addressed.
- Discharge plans and education understood

* Additional information
provided in document text

FIGURE 7.1 FTT management algorithm

- Patient exam must include:
  - Height, weight, head circumference on standard growth
    curve specific for gender, and gestational age
  - Observation of caretaker and infant interaction

– Complete physical exam including evaluation for dysmorphic features
- A list of differential diagnoses was included to aid in the diagnostic evaluation.
- Possible etiologies of failure to thrive include (List by systems adapted from Nelson's Textbook of Pediatrics, Chapter 41, Table 41-3, 20th edition):

  – *Psychosocial/Behavioral*

    Child abuse or neglect
    Child interaction problems (food refusal, autonomy struggles)
    Inadequate diet (poverty, food insufficiency)
    Inadequate food preparation (incorrect mixing of formula)
    Parental or child mental health problems
    Poor parenting skills (lack of knowledge about proper feedings)

  – *Neurological*

    Cerebral palsy
    Neuromuscular or neurodegenerative disorder
    Hypothalamic and other central nervous system tumors (diencephalic syndrome)

  – *Renal*

    Renal failure
    Renal tubular acidosis
    Recurrent urinary tract infection

  – *Endocrine*

    Adrenal insufficiency
    Diabetes insipidus
    Diabetes mellitus
    Growth hormone deficiency
    Thyroid disorder

– *Genetic/Metabolic/Congenital*

> Chromosomal disorders
> Fetal alcohol syndrome
> Inborn errors of metabolism
> Multiple congenital anomaly syndromes (VATER, CHARGE)
> Skeletal dysplasias

– *Gastrointestinal*

> Celiac disease
> Gastroesophageal reflux
> Hirschsprung disease
> Inflammatory bowel disease
> Malabsorption syndromes
> Malrotation
> Milk intolerance
> Pancreatic insufficiency (cystic fibrosis)
> Pyloric stenosis
> Short bowel syndrome
> Food allergy

– *Cardiac*

> Congenital heart disease
> Congestive heart failure
> Vascular rings

– *Pulmonary/Respiratory*

> Bronchopulmonary dysplasia
> Chronic respiratory failure
> Cystic fibrosis
> Obstructive sleep apnea

– *Infectious*

> HIV
> Occult/chronic infections
> Parasitic infections
> Perinatal infections
> Tuberculosis

– *Miscellaneous*

  Collagen vascular disease
  Malignancy
  Primary immunodeficiency

• Malnutrition definition and criteria (Table 7.1)
• Severity and risk assessment, categorized by level of malnutrition and medical instability. Medical instability includes hypothermia defined as a core body temperature below 35 °C (95 °F), bradycardia for age (Table 7.2), hypotension for age (Table 7.3), or significant electrolyte abnormality, e.g., hyponatremia, hypokalemia, and hypernatremia.

TABLE 7.1 Malnutrition definition and criteria

Primary indicators	Mild malnutrition	Moderate malnutrition	Severe malnutrition
Weight for height z-score	−1 to −1.9 z-score	−2 to −2.9 z-score	−3 or greater z-score
BMI for age z-score	−1 to −1.9 z-score	−2 to −2.9 z-score	−3 or greater z-score
Length/height z-score	No data	No data	−3 z-score
Mid-upper arm circumference	≥ −1 to −1.9 z-score	≥ −2 to −2.9 z-score	≥ −3 z-score

Adapted from Aspen Consensus Statement for Identification and Documentation of Pediatric Malnutrition 2015. DOI: 10.1177/0884533614557642

TABLE 7.2 Bradycardia for age (rate/min)

Age	Heart rate
Newborn–5 months	<100
6–11 months	<90
12–48 months	<80

TABLE 7.3 Hypotension for age

Age	Systolic blood pressure
Term neonates (0–28 days)	<60 mmHg
Infants (1–12 months)	<70 mmHg
Children (1–2 years)	<70 mmHg + (age in years ×2) mm Hg

- Admission criteria [6, 18–20]:
  - Medical instability
  - Moderate or severe malnutrition with concern for refeeding syndrome
  - Failed outpatient management
  - Suspected abuse or neglect
  - Concerns about parent–child interaction
  - Risk for loss of follow-up

- Diagnostic evaluation
  - Screening labs and imaging should not be obtained in children with FTT without specific indications identified by history or physical exam. *Evidence Quality: Very low, Recommendation Strength: Strong* [21–23].
  - An upper GI may be obtained in children admitted with FTT and vomiting. *Evidence Quality: Very low, Recommendation Strength: Weak* [1]
  - Screening for refeeding syndrome (basic metabolic profile with magnesium and phosphorus) with appropriate follow-up monitoring may be obtained in children with failure to thrive and moderate or severe malnutrition. Uncomplicated pediatric patients with failure to thrive have a low risk of refeeding syndrome. *Evidence Quality: Low, Recommendation Strength: Weak* [24–26]
  - Review newborn screen
  - If concerns for child abuse: Initiate non-accidental trauma workup. Report to child protective services. Consider Child Abuse Team (CAT) consult.

- Assessment and Monitoring.
  - Daily weights (naked, on the same scale)

- Weekly lengths on a length board
- Strict intake/output documentation (I&Os)
- Record pre- and post-breastfeeding weights
- Caregiver–infant interaction
- OT or speech consult to evaluate feeding technique/ oral-motor assessment.

- Recommended treatments:

    - A multidisciplinary team, consisting of OT (<12 months of age) or speech therapy (≥12 months of age), lactation consultant if breastfeeding, RD, SW, and case management should be involved in the care of pediatric patients admitted for failure to thrive. *Evidence Quality: Weak, Recommendation Strength: Strong* [27–30]
    - A SW evaluation is required for all patients admitted for FTT and a full psychosocial assessment should be performed.
    - Initial diet recommendations (prior to evaluation by nutrition)

        Goal intake of 120 kcal/kg/day
        If 12 mos or older, order appropriate formula or supplement ad lib

    - Consider a multivitamin appropriate for age.
    - Consider 24 h family care demonstration prior to discharge when severe malnutrition on admission assessment or concerns identified by psychosocial assessment.

- Treatments not recommended

    - Labs or imaging without a specific indication identified by history or physical exam *Evidence Quality: Very low, Recommendation Strength: Strong* [21–23]

- Patient and caregiver education:

    - Educational materials regarding the etiology of FTT and the appropriate feeding regimen and/or formula mixing should be given to families and caregivers prior to discharge.

- Discharge criteria and planning:

  - Medical stability (alert and mental status at baseline, hypotension absent, bradycardia absent, hypothermia absent)
  - Labs/imaging are normal or appropriate for outpatient management
  - Appropriate fluid and caloric intake and weight stable or increased
  - Caregiver interaction appropriate or concerns appropriately addressed
  - Caregiver demonstrates appropriate care prior to discharge
  - Discharge plans and education are understood by caregivers
  - Follow-Up: Primary care physician in 1–3 days with an appointment scheduled prior to discharge

- Areas lacking sufficient evidence for a recommendation regarding clinical decision-making were identified as potential areas for research:

  - Do greater z-scores increase the risk for refeeding syndrome?
  - Does 24 h inpatient caregiver care for high-risk families decrease readmission rate?
  - Does monitoring of daily inpatient weights for at least 2 days decrease readmission rate?
  - When should a nasogastric tube be placed if goal calories are not met?

We developed an evidence-based order set to implement the FTT pathway into clinical practice. In addition, we built an FTT Admission History & Physical Exam (H&P) note template to ensure documentation of recommended history and patient exam items. The Malnutrition definition and criteria table (Table 7.1) was included in the note under Assessment as this is unfamiliar to many providers. The reasons for hospital admission such as inadequate response to outpatient management or failed outpatient assessment of psychosocial interaction between child and caregiver were available for providers to select. A notation was included for categorization of FTT as organic versus inorganic. While this terminology is often considered inadequate due to the multifactorial nature of FTT, child protective services in the area surrounding our institution require this documentation whenever involved in a patient's care. Other institutions may or may not find it necessary to include this distinction in an FTT H&P template. Lastly, we created an FTT discharge instruction template including education on etiology of FTT, feeding regimen/diet, and formula mixing.

To capture the improvement in care we hoped to see in our patient population, the following quality metrics were selected:

- Outcomes Measures—hospital length of stay and 30-day readmission rate.
- Process Measures—FTT H&P note usage, documentation of z-scores, order set usage, rate of RD/SW/OT or speech therapy/lactation, and psychology consults ordered
- Balance measure—ED return rate and hospital readmission rate

The pathway was reviewed and approved by the Clinical Pathway Program Steering Committee and implemented in July 2018. An organized and comprehensive plan for rollout with a provider education module was created for pathway adoption. An education slide presentation included how to access the pathway and the associated EMR tools and how to perform certain aspects of patient care such as new or revised feeding procedures (Fig. 7.2). Members of the multidisciplinary team and key stakeholders were tasked with providing education within their area of practice. We encouraged ongoing education to increase and sustain adherence to the pathway.

How Do I Find It?

- Link from the FTT Order Set

- On Anchor → "New Clinical Guidelines site"

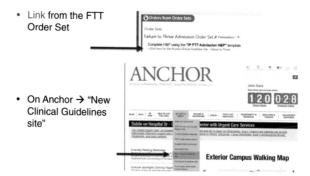

Where do you find the z scores?

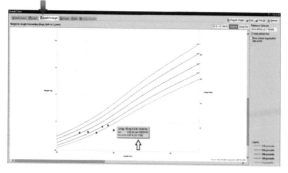

Occupational Therapy

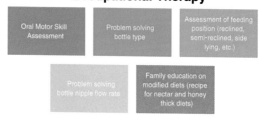

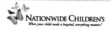

FIGURE 7.2 Examples of provider education slides for pathway rollout

Quality Improvement

General Concepts

After implementation of a pathway, continued QI is important to assure that the standard of care outlined in the pathway is provided as intended. Several QI methods are available, including the Institute for Healthcare Improvement (IHI) PDSA (Plan, Do, Study, Act) model and the Lean/Six Sigma DMAIC (Define, Measure, Analyze, Improve, and Control) model [31, 32]. All models contain similar tools and methodologies. The IHI model was used for the work described in this Case Study.

The team developing a pathway is usually well suited to continue the post rollout QI work. A day-to-day leader should be assigned to serve as the driver of the project. This person assures consistent implementation and data collection.

Defining the Problem

The QI process begins with defining the problem or what the team is trying to accomplish [33]. Areas for improvement can be identified prior to, during, or after development and implementation of the pathway. The aim can be determined through ongoing monitoring of quality metrics, defined prior to or by the pathway. For FTT some teams may choose to address efficiency and resource utilization with aims of reducing the length of stay or readmissions. Other teams may choose to improve multidisciplinary team involvement or certain aspects of care such as rate of daily weight monitoring being performed. A project charter can be used to provide organization for a quality improvement project, aid the team in defining its goal, and in writing the aim of the project.

Measurement

After the charter is in place, the team must perform measurements to determine if change is occurring and if that change is an improvement. Traditional QI measures are outcome measures, process measures, and balancing measures. Outcome measures are those that measure the desired outcome of the QI project. Examples to consider for FTT are length of stay, readmission rate, or resource utilization. Process measures are those that track key steps in the process that lead to the desired change in the outcome measure such as the timely completion of OT/Speech/SW assessments. Balancing measures are those that assess whether the QI work is causing unexpected changes in other areas of the system. For instance, interventions designed to decrease patient length of stay may have the consequence of increasing readmission rates. Decreasing the use of imaging or laboratory tests may adversely affect the diagnostic error rate.

Preliminary data can be displayed in a run chart to show performance of the system over time and to identify early upward or downward trends. When additional data is available, a statistical process control chart (with a defined baseline period and upper and lower control limits) can be created. These limits allow the team to identify the common cause and special cause variation and so differentiate between the normal expected variation inherent to the system and change that is irregular and warrants deeper analysis. In some cases, these instances of special cause variation can be traced to specific QI interventions designed to effect change in the system. At other times they may be an indication of changes in personnel, equipment, methodology, or even hospital census that have had an impact—positively or negatively—on system performance.

We use rules put forth by the American Society for Quality (ASQ) to analyze our data. ASQ defines a process shift as a run of 8 points in a row on the same side of the centerline or 10 of 11 points, 12 of 14, or 16 of 20 points on the same side of the centerline. These rules allow us to account for most of the special cause variation at our institution. There are resources to further explore the rules and uses of run and control charts [34]. In addition to these charts, data analytics software can be used to create dashboards if resources are available. This allows for frequent updates as well as easier analysis and visualization of data.

Problem Analysis

After defining the problem and obtaining baseline data, tools such as cause and effect diagram, 5 why's, process mapping, and key driver diagrams (KDD) can be used for analysis to determine possible root causes for the problem and to direct change ideas [33]. Multidisciplinary team-based generation of ideas or brainstorming of interventions can be high yield. Awareness of an institution's "culture" and reasons why practitioners struggle with changing practice can be important in order to focus on strategies that are more likely to promote change [33, 35, 36]. If an FTT pathway is in place, these strategies can be used to improve adherence to recommended care. Change ideas can be piloted by deploying PDSA rapid cycle small tests of change. When the improvement has been achieved, standardizing the practice and revising the pathway if needed continue to assure stability of improvement and hardwires the change. For guidance, teams may choose to review the Associates in Process Improvement Change concept [37].

Case Study Update

A QI project to decrease the length of stay among patients aged 24 months or less with a primary diagnosis of FTT, malnutrition, or poor weight gain had been started prior to roll out of our FTT pathway. A KDD had initially been created based on a cause and effect analysis (Fig. 7.3) and was subsequently revised after the FTT pathway was implemented (Fig. 7.4).

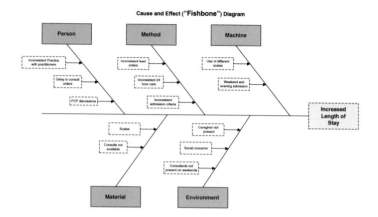

FIGURE 7.3 Cause and effect (Fishbone) diagram for FTT length of stay

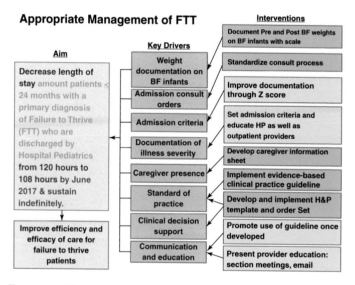

FIGURE 7.4 Key driver diagram for FTT length of stay

A first PDSA cycle aimed to improve the percentage of FTT patients who had diet orders for at least 120 kcal/kg/day (as opposed to ad lib feeding without a defined minimum caloric intake) was initiated. Providers and staff were educated about the intervention and reminders were placed on workroom computers. Diet order data was collected from the EMR to measure compliance with the recommendation and recurrent team feedback was provided. The main barrier encountered during this intervention was maintaining awareness about the new practice each time attendings or residents on service changed.

After the FTT pathway was implemented, the KDD was updated with an ancillary services bundle, including RD, OT/Speech, and SW consults ordered within 2 h of admission to the hospital unit. As these orders were included in the new pathway order set, the second PDSA focused on increasing pathway order set use. Bundle and order set compliance were analyzed in control charts as well as by visualization software and eventually included in an FTT dashboard. The main barrier to adherence for PDSA cycle 2 was low resident awareness about the pathway order set so recurrent education and reminders were instituted. Additional PDSAs were done to increase FTT H&P template usage, malnutrition severity documentation, pre- and post-breastfeeding weights entry into the EMR, and rate of caregivers receiving the FTT discharge education handout.

Lessons Learned and Future Directions

- An FTT pathway for hospitalized infants and young children should be developed by a multidisciplinary team applying evidence-based methodology and incorporating appropriate clinical support tools. Pathway implementation is best combined with a series of quality improvement initiatives to improve quality and value of care.
- An appropriate next step of the work described here is to extend the pathway to expand on recommendations in the outpatient setting, with the goal of optimizing care and decreasing the need for hospitalization.

Acknowledgments The pathway development process described in this chapter was supported by experts at the Evidence-Based Outcomes Center (EBOC) at Texas Children's Hospital and was developed in collaboration with the Pediatric Initiative for Clinical Standards (PICS).

References

1. Larson-Nath C, St Clair N, Goday P. Hospitalization for failure to thrive: a prospective descriptive report. Clin Pediatr (Phila). 2018;57(2):212–9.
2. Lawal AK, Rotter T, Kinsman L, Machotta A, Ronellenfitsch U, Scott SD, et al. What is a clinical pathway? Refinement of an operational definition to identify clinical pathway studies for a Cochrane systematic review. BMC Med. 2016;14:35.
3. Clinical Standard Work Pathways and Tools: @seattlechildren; 2020. Available from https://www.seattlechildrens.org/healthcare-professionals/gateway/clinical-resources/pathways/
4. Clinical Pathways Program. Children's Hospital of Philadelphia 2020. Available from https://www.chop.edu/pathways
5. Clinical Standards. Texas Children's Hospital 2020. Available from https://www.texaschildrens.org/departments/safety-outcomes/clinical-standards
6. Olsen EM, Petersen J, Skovgaard AM, Weile B, Jørgensen T, Wright CM. Failure to thrive: the prevalence and concurrence of anthropometric criteria in a general infant population. Arch Dis Child. 2007;92(2):109–14.
7. Argyle J. Approaches to detecting growth faltering in infancy and childhood. Ann Hum Biol. 2003;30(5):499–519.
8. Shah MD. Failure to thrive in children. J Clin Gastroenterol. 2002;35(5):371–4.
9. Prevention CfDCa. WHO growth standards are recommended for use in the U.S. for infants and children 0 to 2 years of age 2010. Available from https://www.cdc.gov/growthcharts/who_charts.htm#The%20WHO%20Growth%20Charts
10. Prevention CfDCa. Clinical growth charts 2017. Available from https://www.cdc.gov/growthcharts/clinical_charts.htm#Set1
11. Guyatt G, Oxman AD, Akl EA, Kunz R, Vist G, Brozek J, et al. GRADE guidelines: 1. Introduction-GRADE evidence profiles and summary of findings tables. J Clin Epidemiol. 2011;64(4):383–94.

12. de Onis M, Onyango AW, Borghi E, Siyam A, Nishida C, Siekmann J. Development of a WHO growth reference for school-aged children and adolescents. Bull World Health Organ. 2007;85(9):660–7.

13. Olsen EM. Failure to thrive: still a problem of definition. Clin Pediatr (Phila). 2006;45(1):1–6.

14. GOMEZ F, GALVAN RR, CRAVIOTO J, FRENK S. Malnutrition in infancy and childhood, with special reference to kwashiorkor. Adv Pediatr. 1955;7:131–69.

15. Waterlow JC. Classification and definition of protein-calorie malnutrition. Br Med J. 1972;3(5826):566–9.

16. Waterlow JC, Buzina R, Keller W, Lane JM, Nichaman MZ, Tanner JM. The presentation and use of height and weight data for comparing the nutritional status of groups of children under the age of 10 years. Bull World Health Organ. 1977;55(4):489–98.

17. Grover Z, Ee LC. Protein energy malnutrition. Pediatr Clin North Am. 2009;56(5):1055–68.

18. Jaffe AC. Failure to thrive: current clinical concepts. Pediatr Rev. 2011;32(3):100–7. quiz 8

19. Careaga MG, Kerner JA. A gastroenterologist's approach to failure to thrive. Pediatr Ann. 2000;29(9):558–67.

20. Hren I, Mis NF, Brecelj J, Campa AS, Sedmak M, Krzisnik C, et al. Effects of formula supplementation in breast-fed infants with failure to thrive. Pediatr Int. 2009;51(3):346–51.

21. Sills RH. Failure to thrive. The role of clinical and laboratory evaluation. Am J Dis Child. 1978;132(10):967–9.

22. Berwick DM, Levy JC, Kleinerman R. Failure to thrive: diagnostic yield of hospitalisation. Arch Dis Child. 1982;57(5):347–51.

23. Homer C, Ludwig S. Categorization of etiology of failure to thrive. Am J Dis Child. 1981;135(9):848–51.

24. Afzal NA, Addai S, Fagbemi A, Murch S, Thomson M, Heuschkel R. Refeeding syndrome with enteral nutrition in children: a case report, literature review and clinical guidelines. Clin Nutr. 2002;21(6):515–20.

25. Boateng AA, Sriram K, Meguid MM, Crook M. Refeeding syndrome: treatment considerations based on collective analysis of literature case reports. Nutrition. 2010;26(2):156–67.

26. Friedli N, Stanga Z, Sobotka L, Culkin A, Kondrup J, Laviano A, et al. Revisiting the refeeding syndrome: results of a systematic review. Nutrition. 2017;35:151–60.

27. Wright CM, Callum J, Birks E, Jarvis S. Effect of community based management in failure to thrive: randomised controlled trial. BMJ. 1998;317(7158):571–4.
28. Hobbs C, Hanks HG. A multidisciplinary approach for the treatment of children with failure to thrive. Child Care Health Dev. 1996;22(4):273–84.
29. Bithoney WG, McJunkin J, Michalek J, Snyder J, Egan H, Epstein D. The effect of a multidisciplinary team approach on weight gain in nonorganic failure-to-thrive children. J Dev Behav Pediatr. 1991;12(4):254–8.
30. Atalay A, McCord M. Characteristics of failure to thrive in a referral population: implications for treatment. Clin Pediatr (Phila). 2012;51(3):219–25.
31. Institute for Healthcare Improvement. Available from http://www.ihi.org/
32. Lean Six Sigma Institute. Certification & Implementation Services 2020. Available from https://www.leansixsigmainstitute.org
33. Ogrinc G. Fundamentals of health care improvement: a guide to improving your patients' care. 3rd ed. Joint Commission Resources; 2020.
34. Control chart—statistical process control charts. ASQ 2020. Available from https://asq.org/quality-resources/control-chart
35. Kotter J. John Kotter: updated 8 step process of change 2020. Available from https://www.change-management-coach.com/john-kotter.html
36. Langley GJ. The improvement guide: a practical approach to enhancing organizational performance. 2nd ed; 2020.
37. API—Associates in Process Improvement—Home 2020. Available from https://www.apiweb.org/

Index

© Springer Nature Switzerland AG 2023   169
J. G. Vachani (ed.), *Failure to Thrive and Malnutrition*,
https://doi.org/10.1007/978-3-031-14164-5

Printed in the United States
by Baker & Taylor Publisher Services